Frontiers in Anti-Cancer Drug Discovery

(Volume 8)

Edited by

Atta-ur-Rahman, *FRS*
Kings College, University of Cambridge, Cambridge, UK

M. Iqbal Choudhary
H.E.J. Research Institute of Chemistry, International Center for Chemical and Biological Sciences, University of Karachi, Karachi, Pakistan

General:

1. Any dispute or claim arising out of or in connection with this License Agreement or the Work (including non-contractual disputes or claims) will be governed by and construed in accordance with the laws of the U.A.E. as applied in the Emirate of Dubai. Each party agrees that the courts of the Emirate of Dubai shall have exclusive jurisdiction to settle any dispute or claim arising out of or in connection with this License Agreement or the Work (including non-contractual disputes or claims).
2. Your rights under this License Agreement will automatically terminate without notice and without the need for a court order if at any point you breach any terms of this License Agreement. In no event will any delay or failure by Bentham Science Publishers in enforcing your compliance with this License Agreement constitute a waiver of any of its rights.
3. You acknowledge that you have read this License Agreement, and agree to be bound by its terms and conditions. To the extent that any other terms and conditions presented on any website of Bentham Science Publishers conflict with, or are inconsistent with, the terms and conditions set out in this License Agreement, you acknowledge that the terms and conditions set out in this License Agreement shall prevail.

Bentham Science Publishers Ltd.
Executive Suite Y - 2
PO Box 7917, Saif Zone
Sharjah, U.A.E.
Email: subscriptions@benthamscience.org

BENTHAM SCIENCE

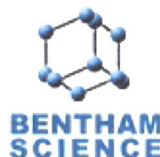

CONTENTS

Preface

Cancer is a grand health challenge of modern times, being the second leading cause of death. Despite tremendous investments in this field, the prognosis of cancer has not improved substantially. There have been some advances in cancer chemotherapy and radiation therapy, but other treatment options, such as surgery, burn, immunotherapy, *etc* remain primitive and far from being perfect. Chemotherapy, the "holy grail" of cancer treatment, is based on targeting certain biomolecular pathways in the complex cascade of cancer progression. However, the limited understanding of cancer biology often makes this a *fishing expedition*. As a result, many of the currently available anti-cancer drugs are non-specific and less effective. Heterogenicities in cancer pheno- and geno-types, often make the identification of genuine targets difficult. However recent advancements in genomics, metabolomics, transcriptomics, and molecular biology have fuelled major research projects in the fields of oncology and anti-cancer drug discovery and development. The scientific literature is now full of exciting discoveries against this disease of modern society, cancer. It is often difficult, even for a prolific reader, to keep pace with these developments. Thus, the need of a comprehensive book review series is greatly felt.

The last seven volumes of the *ebook* series "*Frontiers in Anti-Cancer Drug Discovery*" have attracted major interest, making this series a welcome addition to the global literature on this dynamic topic. The present 8th volume of this internationally recognized books series comprises six carefully selected topics focused on various aspects of cancer chemotherapy and cancer biology, contributed by leading experts in this field. Each chapter deals with anti-cancer drug discovery and development based on various innovative approaches, including identification of new molecular targets, manipulation of cancer microenvironment, and outcomes of pre-clinical and clinical studies on new drugs, and combination therapies.

Amedei *et al.* have reviewed the recent progress in the use various immunotherapies in cancer treatment in chapter 1. Their emphasis is on the treatment of gastrointestinal cancers by T-cell based immunotherapies. T-Cells, also called T-lymphocytes, are a subtype of white blood cells that play a central role in cell-mediated immunity. T-Cell based immunotherapies have attracted considerable scientific attention. However, T-cell based immunotherapy of cancers is not free of adverse side effects.

In chapter 2, Cheng *et al.* have contributed a comprehensive review on the anticancer activity of the newly discovered compound adjudin, a well-known male reversible contraceptive used in animals. Adjudin is a structural analogue of the anticancer drug lonidamine. Apart from its known potent anti-spermatogenic activities, adjudin is found to have many other biological properties. Notable among them is its activity against neuroinflammation, protection against gentamicin-induced ototoxicity, and prevention of cancer growth and development. The authors have critically reviewed the recent literature on new indications of this old contraceptive drug. The focus of the article is on recently discovered anticancer activities of adjudin, either alone or in combination with other anticancer drugs as well as with nanocarriers. Adjudin, similar to lonidamine, inhibit cancer growth by targeting mitochondria and blocking energy metabolism in certain kinds of tumor cells in mice, indicating that it is potential anticancer agent.

Tumor microenvironment (TME) plays an important role in the progression of tumor growth, and treatment outcome. This cellular environment includes surrounding blood vessels, immune cells, fibroblasts, bone marrow-derived inflammatory cells, lymphocytes, signalling molecules and the extracellular matrix (ECM). Recently TME has been identified as potential target for novel cancer chemotherapies. Mabtel and Pepper have contributed a comprehensive review in chapter 3 on the role of tumor microenvironment in tumor progression, angiogenesis, cellular invasion, metastatic dissemination, resistance against chemotherapy and its potential as drug target. Recently developed treatments which can modulate TME against tumor growth, along with their mechanisms of action, have also been discussed.

In chapter 4, Fatima *et al.* have focussed on the current and emerging therapies for the treatment of hepatocellular carcinoma (HCC) or malignant hepatoma. Hepatocellular carcinoma accounts for most liver cancers, and is a leading cause of cancer related deaths. HCC occurs more frequently in men than women and is usually diagnosed in people of age 50 or older. HCC's prognosis is among the poorest of all cancer types. This review provides a detailed description of various treatment options for HCC, and their advantages and disadvantages. Future directions of development in this field are also reviewed.

Gold complexes are known for a variety of biological activities. In chapter 5 Sun *et al.* discuss the anti-cancer properties of gold-based compounds and their potential. After the serendipitous discovery of cisplatin, a platinum (II) based compound, as a potent anti-cancer agent, interest in metal complexes has increased exponentially. Sun *et al.* have critically reviewed the recent literature on the therapeutic potential of novel gold complexes (I and III), particularly against various cancers.

In the last chapter, Anreddy *et al.* have reviewed the application of nanostructures as oral drug delivery vehicles for the treatment of various cancers. One of the key issues in cancer chemotherapy is that the most potent anticancer therapies can only be administered through injection, as their oral drug delivery is associated with many limitations. This makes cancer chemotherapy quite challenging. Recently many new classes of nanoparticles (NPs), such as liposomes, polymeric NPs, polymeric conjugates, micelles, dendrimers, polymersomes, and metallic and inorganic NPs, have been developed as new drug delivery vehicles for oral administration in cancer chemotherapy. These nanoparticle-based anti-cancer drugs are often devoid of problems such as poor solubility, low intrinsic permeability, and metabolic changes. The potential of NPs in on-target and sustained administration of drugs is also discussed.

We wish to express our sincere gratitude to all the authors for their excellent scholarly contributions to this 8th volume of this book series. We also appreciate the efforts of the impressive production team of Bentham Science Publishers for the efficient processing the treatise. The efforts of Ms. Fariya Zulfiqar (Assistant Manager Publications) & Mr. Shehzad Naqvi (Senior Manager Publications) and excellent management of Mr. Mahmood Alam (Director Publications) are greatly appreciated. We also hope that like the previous volumes of this internationally recognized book series, the current volume will also receive wide readership and recognition.

Atta-ur-Rahman, *FRS*
Kings College
University of Cambridge
UK

M. Iqbal Choudhary
H.E.J. Research Institute of Chemistry
International Center for Chemical and
Biological Sciences
University of Karachi, Pakistan

List of Contributors

Albert S.-C. Chan Guangzhou Lee & Man Technology Company Limited, Nansha, Guangzhou, China

Amedeo Amedei Department of Experimental and Clinical Medicine, University of Florence, 350134 Florence, Italy

Bruno Silvestrini S.B.M. Srl Pharmaceuticals, Rome, Italy

C. Yan Cheng The Mary M. Wohlford Laboratory for Male Contraceptive Research, Center for Biomedical Research, Population Council, 1230 York Ave, New York, USA

Carolina V. De Almeida Department of Experimental and Clinical Medicine, University of Florence, 350134 Florence, Italy

Chih-Chiang Chen Guangzhou Lee & Man Technology Company Limited, Nansha, Guangzhou, China

Chunxia Chen Guangzhou Lee & Man Technology Company Limited, Nansha, Guangzhou, China

Dolores Mruk The Mary M. Wohlford Laboratory for Male Contraceptive Research, Center for Biomedical Research, Population Council, 1230 York Ave, New York, USA

Elizabeth Tang The Mary M. Wohlford Laboratory for Male Contraceptive Research, Center for Biomedical Research, Population Council, 1230 York Ave, New York, USA

Haiqi Chen The Mary M. Wohlford Laboratory for Male Contraceptive Research, Center for Biomedical Research, Population Council, 1230 York Ave, New York, USA

Chih-Chiang Chen Guangzhou Lee & Man Technology Company Limited, Nansha, Guangzhou, China

Mahendar Porika Department of Biotechnology, Kakatiya University, Warangal, 506009, India

Man-Kin Tse Guangzhou Lee & Man Technology Company Limited, Nansha, Guangzhou, Guangdong, P.R. China

Michael S. Pepper Institute for Cellular and Molecular Medicine, Department of Immunology, and SAMRC Extramural Unit for Stem Cell Research and Therapy, Faculty of Health Sciences, University of Pretoria, South Africa

Nikki P. Lee Department of Surgery, The University of Hong Kong, Pokfulam, Hong Kong SAR, China

Peace Mabeta Angiogenesis Laboratory, Department of Physiology, Faculty of Health Sciences, University of Pretoria, South Africa

Qing Wen The Mary M. Wohlford Laboratory for Male Contraceptive Research, Center for Biomedical Research, Population Council, 1230 York Ave, New York, USA

Radhika Tippani Department of Biotechnology, Kakatiya University, Warangal, 506009, India

Rama Narsimha Reddy Anreddy Department of Pharmacology, Jyothishmathi Institute of Pharmaceutical Sciences, Ramakrishna Colony, Thimmapur, Karimnagar 505481, India

Ramon Kaneno Department of Microbiology and Immunology, Institute of Biosciences – São Paulo State University, 18618-610, Botucatu, SP, Brazil

Raymond Wai-Yin Sun	Department of Chemistry, Shantou University, 243 Daxue Road, Shantou, China Guangzhou Lee & Man Technology Company Limited, Nansha, Guangzhou, China Department of Chemistry, The University of Hong Kong, Pokfulam Road, Hong Kong
Srividya Lonkala	Department of Pharmacology, Jyothishmathi Institute of Pharmaceutical Sciences, Ramakrishna Colony, Thimmapur, Karimnagar 505481, India
Sarwat Fatima	Lab of Brain and Gut Research, Centre of Clinical Research for Chinese Medicine, School of Chinese Medicine, Hong Kong Baptist University, Kowloon Tong, China Centre for Cancer and Inflammation Research, School of Chinese Medicine, Hong Kong Baptist University, Kowloon Tong, China
Weiliang Xia	State Key Laboratory of Oncogenes and Related Genes, Renji-Med X Stem Cell Research Center, Ren Ji Hospital; School of Biomedical Engineering, Shanghai Jiao Tong University, Shanghai, China
Xiang Xiao	The Mary M. Wohlford Laboratory for Male Contraceptive Research, Center for Biomedical Research, Population Council, 1230 York Ave, New York, USA Department of Reproductive Physiology, Zhejiang Academy of Medical Sciences, Hangzhou 310013, China
Yan-ho Cheng	The Mary M. Wohlford Laboratory for Male Contraceptive Research, Center for Biomedical Research, Population Council, 1230 York Ave, New York, USA Oncology and Hematology Program, Department of Medicine, Westchester Medical Center, Valhalla, USA
Ying Gao	The Mary M. Wohlford Laboratory for Male Contraceptive Research, Center for Biomedical Research, Population Council, 1230 York Ave, New York, USA
Zhao Xiang Bian	Lab of Brain and Gut Research, Centre of Clinical Research for Chinese Medicine, School of Chinese Medicine, Hong Kong Baptist University, Kowloon Tong, China Centre for Cancer and Inflammation Research, School of Chinese Medicine, Hong Kong Baptist University, Kowloon Tong, China

CHAPTER 1

T Cells in Gastrointestinal Cancers: Role and Therapeutic Strategies

Carolina V. De Almeida[1], Ramon Kaneno[2] and Amedeo Amedei[1,*]

[1] Department of Experimental and Clinical Medicine, University of Florence, 350134 Florence, Italy

[2] Department of Microbiology and Immunology, Institute of Biosciences – São Paulo State University, 18618-610, Botucatu, SP, Brazil

Abstract: Conventional treatments of gastrointestinal cancers based on surgical resection and chemotherapy are not enough to eradicate potentially relapsing tumor cells and can also impair the immune system functions. Immunotherapies aim to help the body to eradicate cancer and other diseases, by modulating the immune system. They can be performed by active approaches, usually orchestrated by dendritic cell vaccines that present a specific tumor associated antigen to T cells, or passive approaches, which have the T cells as protagonist, and are based on antitumor antibodies, or adoptive cell transfer. T lymphocyte subsets can exhibit different role face to a tumor scenario, varying from an effective cellular antitumor response to a regulatory participation. Although a lot of protocols to combat cancer progression have been proposed, T cell-based immunotherapies in gastrointestinal cancers are still not approved for clinical applications mainly because of their side effects. Nowadays, promising protocols combining two or more approaches, aiming to create an efficient therapy without or with fewer side effects. In this chapter, we made a review about the role of T cells on cancer, especially focusing on gastrointestinal cancer immunotherapeutic methods.

Keywords: Adoptive immunotherapy, Gastrointestinal cancer, Immunotherapy, Infiltrating lymphocyte, Tumor lymphocyte engineering, T lymphocytes.

INTRODUCTION

Gastrointestinal (GI) cancers, including colorectal (CRC), gastric, pancreatic, liver and bile duct cancers, are complex diseases that figure among the ten most frequent types of cancers annually diagnosed worldwide [1], which incidences have a variable geographic distribution [2]. Most of these tumors occur in a sporadic way, and the distribution variability is closely associated with diet

* **Corresponding author Amedeo Amedei:** Department of Experimental and Clinical Medicine, University of Florence, 350134 Florence, Italy; Tel: +39 055 2758330; E-mail: amedeo.amedei@unifi.it

Atta-ur-Rahman & M. Iqbal Choudhary (Eds.)

culture and lifestyle [3 - 6]. The development of GI cancers could also be associated with microbial infections, which seems to play an important role on both, initiation and progression. For instance, *Streptococcus bovis* is an important inducer of CRC development [7], while *Helicobacter pylori* is highly associated with gastric cancer [8], and the Hepatitis C virus induces liver cancer [9]. The association of these pathogens with previously stabilized chronic inflammatory microenvironment can induce DNA damage in proliferating cells through the action of reactive oxygen species (ROS) and inflammatory cytokines that can culminate in gene mutations and/or epigenetic changes [10].

Conventional treatment of patients with localized GI cancers consists in surgical resection of tumor tissue. However, post-surgery relapsing disease frequently develops within 2 years in approximately 40% of patients. Therefore, adjuvant therapy is required to improve anti-cancer responsiveness in high-risk patients, and then, surgery is usually followed by adjuvant chemotherapy or adjuvant chemo-radiotherapy. Frequently, patients are submitted to perioperative chemotherapy [11, 12] (also called neoadjuvant therapy administrated before surgery), in order to reduce the tumor mass and facilitate surgical intervention. Despite these combinations, metastasis and relapsing diseases are until the main causes of death in GI patients. Moreover, *in vitro* and *in vivo* studies have shown that cytotoxic chemotherapy, as well as the surgery stress itself, can impair the immu-nological steady state and also the ability to develop an antitumor immune res-ponse [13].

The immune system plays an important role in the battle against cancer development. The capacity to promote an effective immunological reaction against tumor antigens was firstly described by Macfarlane Burnet and Lewis Thomas and called immunosurveillance [14]. Immunosurveillance occurs when some antigens, encoded by mutated genes and expressed by tumor cells, became a functional target and are quickly recognized and destroyed by innate effector cells such as natural killer cells. This concept of surveillance can be extended to recognition, processing, and presentation of tumor antigens by professional antigen-presenting cells (APCs) to *naïve* lymphocytes (Ly) [15, 16]. In this scenario, autologous CD4+ and CD8+ T lymphocytes recognize these antigens, and attack transformed cells inducing their lysis [17]. In fact, the presence of strong lymphocyte infiltration in tumor site such as in melanoma, CRC and ovarian cancers is associated with a good clinical outcome, since they have the function to inhibit the tumor growth [18].

Lymphocytes originate from a common lymphoid precursor cell in bone marrow. During fetal development, some of these lymphoid precursors move to thymic epithelium to develop this organ where all T lymphocytes will evolve (Fig. **1**). T cells have surface receptors (TCRs) that recognize antigen peptide linked to molecules of the Major Histocompatibility Complex (MHC), especially expressed on the surface of the APCs such as macrophage and dendritic cells (DC), or also on the target cells, such as allogeneic cells and virus or intracellular bacterial - infected cells.

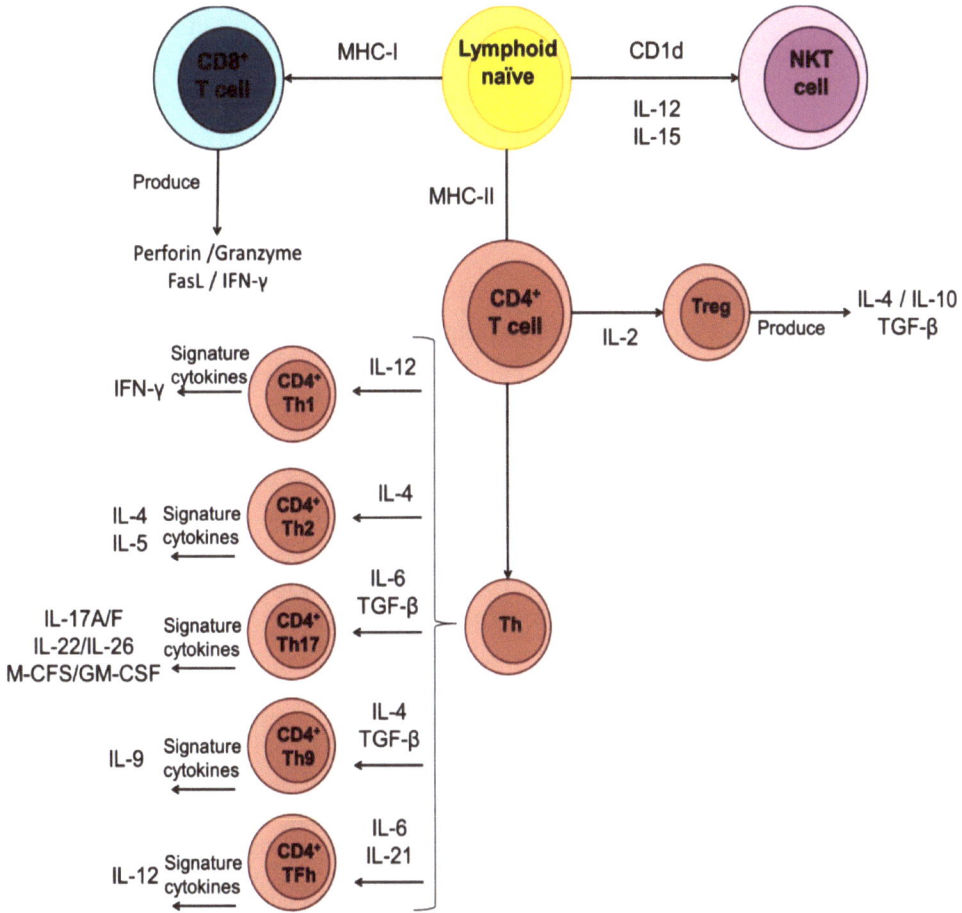

Fig. (1). T lymphocytes' differentiation: from the common progenitor to the different subpopulations CD8, CD4 and Natural killer T lymphocytes (NKT). When a naïve lymphocyte recognizes an antigen, which was presented by a major histocompatibility complex class I (MHC-I) is induced to differentiate to a CD8$^+$ profile. However, the recognition of antigen presented by MHC-II in turn, guides the lymphocytes' differentiation for a CD4$^+$ subpopulation, which after activation may enter several different pathways depending on antigen-presenting cell (APC) co-stimulatory factors and cytokine setting. The presence of Interleukin (IL)-12, for example, directs the CD4$^+$ to Th (T helper) -1 profile, while IL-4 to Th2, IL-6 and TGF-β to Th17, IL-4 and TGF-β to Th9, IL-6 and IL-21 to T follicular helper (TFh) cells and finally, the presence of IL-2 conducts the CD4$^+$ T lymphocytes to differentiate in T regulatory (Treg) cells. The differentiation of NKT cells in the other hand occurs when naïve T lymphocytes recognize CD1d in the presence of IL-12 and IL-15.

TCR are heterodimers composed of two polypeptide chains, usually α and β, that show a constant (C) and a variable (V) regions. The V region presents three hypervariable regions called Complementary Determining Regions (CDR), which are responsible for the recognition of the peptide-MHC complex. Those T lymphocytes CD4[+] can recognize peptides linked to class II MHC molecules, while those CD8[+] link the peptides which are complexed with MHC class I molecules. After the peptide recognition, CD4 and CD8 molecules link to a non-polymorphic region of MHC molecules to stabilize the TCR-MHC association and then signalize for the T cell activation. Lymphocytes also express accessory molecules that take part in antigen-induced cell activation, such as CD2, CD11a, CD28, CD40 ligand [19]. Besides the regular αβ polypeptide receptors, there is a low percentage of T cells with TCR formed by γ and δ chains (Tγδ), whose features will be discussed further.

The CD4[+], also called *T helpers (Th)*, have the role of helping the others cells of the immune system in their function, such as B lymphocytes, macrophage, NK cells and other T Ly, producing cytokines responsible for their activation (Fig. **2A**). The T helper lymphocytes are classified as Th1, Th2, Th17, Th9 and Tfh according to their functions and with the secreted cytokines (Fig. **1**). The Th1 lymphocytes, for example, produce high levels of IFN-γ and drive immune system towards to a cellular response. This reactivity is characterized by activation of macrophages and cytotoxic T cells that evolve to an effective response against intracellular bacteria and virus. This responsiveness is also essential for the acute rejection of allografts [20], and is the most important for resistance to tumor cell [21]. Moreover, the development of CD8[+] T lymphocytes depends on the Th1 profile immune response activation [22].

The Th2 cell subset is responsible to produce IL-4, IL-5, IL-10 and IL-13, and its immune response toward polarization results in high levels of IgE, improving the immunity against extracellular parasites as well as, can determinate type I hypersensitivity. Interleukins produced by Th2 lymphocytes have a strong negative regulatory role of Th1 cells, therefore the prevalence of Th2 responsiveness is associated with effectiveness delays of antitumor defenses [23].

Secreted by Th17 lymphocytes, the IL-17, IL-21 and IL-22 cytokines lead to an immune response towards to inflammatory reactions. Then, although inflammation is an innate reaction of the body against aggressors, it can also be triggered as a consequence of a specific immune response. This defense reaction is particularly relevant in fungal and extracellular bacterial infections responses [24], however, it is strongly associated with auto-inflammatory diseases, such as autoimmune arthritis [25], and Crohn´s disease [26]. The negative influence of Th17 on tumor development deserves special attention in CRC, since inflammation is one of the main predisposing factors of this cancer type development. In fact, while administration of non-steroidal anti-inflammatory drugs helps to control the cancer growth [27], the recruitment of Th17 lymphocytes is associated with enhancement of the CRC development [28].

Follicular helper T cells (Tfh), which help B lymphocytes at lymphoid follicles, produce IL-21 and seem to be derived from Th2 lymphocytes [29, 30]. In fact, some human Tfh cells express the Th2 marker CRTH2 and can also produce IL-4 [31]. Another subset that seems to result from the Th2 plasticity is referred as Th9 cells, a population that switches the production of IL-4 to IL-9 upon stimulation with TGF-β [32]. Similarly to Th2, Th9 also takes part in anti-helm-intic response and allergic reaction [33, 34].

The functions of these T helper cell subsets are regulated by immunosuppressive cells named regulatory T cells (Treg), which comprise heterogeneous subpopulations with phenotypical and functional particularities, but sharing common features such as the expression of CD4 and the α chain receptor for IL-2 (CD25) [35, 36]. Transcription factor Forkhead Box P3 (FoxP3) is also used to identify Treg, although subsets called Tr1 and Th3 do not have this factor (FoxP3- subsets) [37].

The CD8+ T cells usually evolve to effector cytolytic T lymphocytes (CTL) (Fig. **2B**). These cells have cytoplasmic granules full of perforin monomers, granzyme and granulysin that are released at the intercellular pouch formed between effector and target cell membranes after the target recognition by the CTL [38]. Perforin monomers polymerize on target cell membranes, forming transmembrane pores on this surface, allowing the cytoplasmic content leaking, the influx of hypotonic extracellular liquid, and consequently the osmotic lysis [39]. In addition, these perforin-formed pores permit the release of granzyme into the target cells triggering the cell apoptosis [40], that is induced by the DNA break, which can be caused by diverse pathways such as the induction of caspase activation, mito-chondrial impairment, and nuclear disruption [41, 42].

Therefore, CD8+ CTL are classically considered the main antitumor effector cells, since they recognize tumor antigens in a HLA ABC-restricted manner, show clonal expansion, and their effectiveness could be improved including immuno-logical memory [43]. However, their activation and evolution into cytolytic antitumor cells improve the antitumor status [44].

Other immune cells that are involved in the immune response against cancer are the natural killer (NK) and the natural killer T cells (NKT). NK cells are circulating lymphocytes able to extravasate and infiltrate different tissues containing malignant cells [45, 46]. Most natural killer activity is attributed to a population of cells morphologically defined as large granular lymphocytes (LGL), found in peripheral blood and lymphoid organs [47 - 49]. These cells are larger than typical small lymphocytes, with higher cytoplasm: nucleus ratio and large azurophilic cytoplasm granules [50].

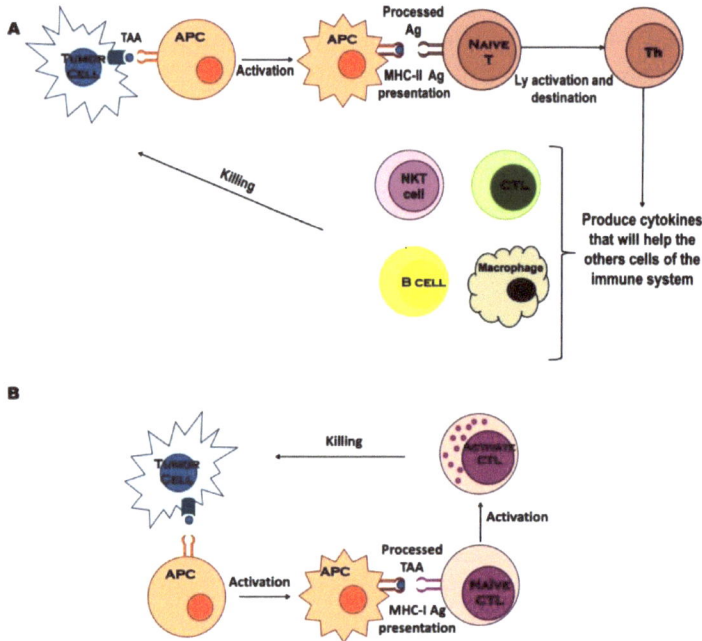

Fig. (2). CD4$^+$ and CD8$^+$ T cells' activation by tumor cells. A) Tumor associated antigens (TAA) are presented by an antigen-presenting cell (APC) through the major histocompatibility complex class II (MHC-II) to a naïve lymphocyte. After recognizing this antigen, the naïve T lymphocyte becomes a mature CD4$^+$ or also named as T helper lymphocyte (Th), and start to produce cytokines that will help other cells of the immune system, such as macrophages, CD8$^+$, Natural killer T lymphocytes (NKT) and lymphocyte B, to execute their functions. B) In a second way, antigens derived from endogenous peptides are presented to the naïve T lymphocyte by the APC through MHC-I, managing it differentiation to a cytotoxic T lymphocyte (CTL-CD8$^+$) profile, which will produce cytotoxic granulates such as granzymes, perforin, and granulysin able to induce tumor cell apoptosis.

NK cells comprise 10-15% of all circulating lymphocytes, but can also be found in peripheral tissues such as liver, peritoneal cavity, lung and placenta. They are usually present in a standby state in the peripheral blood, but after their activation by specific cytokines, they become capable of extravasation and infiltration into most infected tissues or the tumor site [51]. These cells are potent effectors of the innate immune system, since they have a critical role in early host defense against invading intracellular pathogens [52], and for their ability to kill virus-infected and cancer cells [53], are suitable candidates for immunotherapy of both hemato-logic and solid tumors [54].

As previously reviewed by Kaneno R, since NK do not express CD3, TCR or any other TCR chains (α, β, γ or δ), nor even B lymphocyte markers CD19 and surface Ig, these cells are classified as non-T, non-B lymphocytes. Although these cells share the CD16 expression with macrophages and neutrophils, they are non-adherent leukocytes and do not show phagocytic activity [46].

They constitute a phenotypically heterogeneous population with a variety of surface markers involved in antigen recognition, lytic activity triggering and cell regulation [55 - 57]. Among them, NKG2D is the main activation C-type lectin-like receptor that binds to DAP-10 adaptor molecule that triggers tumor cell lysis [58]. NKG2D interacts with MIC A and MIC B, homologous to class I structures that conserve the domains α1, α2 and α3 of class I MHC molecules, but fail to express both β2-microglobulin and peptides bound to the α chain [59]. MIC A and MIC B are uncommon on normal cells while epithelial tumor cells express them in a high density, being important targets for NK [57, 60, 61]. After the interaction between effector and target cells, immunological synapses are formed between the cell surfaces and NK cells release the contents of cytoplasmic granules, as previously described for CTL.

Although experimental data have shown that NK activity can be important to inhibit the occurrence of colon cancer metastasis, their efficiency in the immuno-surveillance of this cancer type in humans cannot be very easily demonstrable. Although CRC shows a low number of infiltrating NK cells [62, 63], their presence is associated with a better prognosis for patients not only with CRC [64], but also with gastric carcinoma [65].

The NK cells of CRC patients show the same level of lytic activity from normal donors, however, the cells isolated from tumor tissue have a reduced lytic activity when compared with NK cells of peripheral blood or mucosa-associated lymphoid tissue of the same patient [66]. This is in agreement with the local suppressive environment, induced by suppressive factors produced by the tumor cells themselves, associated with a strong Treg activity in gastrointestinal tissue.

Tissues obtained from metastasis also show reduced frequency or even absence of NK cells, whereas patients submitted to treatment with cytokines show a marked increase in these effector cells (CD56$^+$/CD3$^-$), in the adjacent tumor [67]. Considering that NK activity results from the balance between stimulatory and inhibitory signals, it must be remembered that, similar to other regulatory systems, inhibitory signals are more potent than the simulated ones. So, in some conditions NK cells require additional stimulation by cytokines, whose *in vivo* production can improve the defensive role of these cells [68].

NKT cells recognize, and share phenotypic and functional properties common to both conventional NK cells and T cells [69]. They are able to induce tumor cell death by producing cell-death-inducing effectors molecules such as perforins, FasL, TRAIL, IFN-γ and IL-4 [70, 71]. NKT cells are a group of lymphocytes that express both, TCR and NK markers, and recognize lipid antigens (mainly glycolipids and glycerols) presented by the class Ib molecule, CD1d, differently from conventional T cells that recognize protein (peptide) antigens presented by MHC molecules. They are an important immunoregulatory cell subset activated during the immune differentiation towards Th1 or Th2, and are key tags in several studies, including transplantation, tumors, autoimmunity and allergy [72, 73].

Mucous, enterocytes, and the bowel wall work as physical innate barriers of gastrointestinal system to pathogens. When they fail, gut can be infiltrated by phagocytic cells, such as neutrophils and macrophages, followed by activation of inflammatory and complement pathways [74]. Inflammatory process aims to destroy pathogens and abnormal tissues, and is responsible for promoting tissue reconstruction. However, in the cancer scenario, this inflammatory process is rather associated with the carcinogenesis promotion, especially for the secretion of several cytokines and growth factors with carcinogenic activity as TNF [75], IL-8 [76], VEGF [77]. Thus, increased density of microvessel density, as well as maintenance of the inflammatory response is associated with poor survival and enhancement of cancer growth. An example of inflammation pro-carcinogenic role in CRC includes the strong association with chronic inflammatory diseases such as Crohn's disease and ulcerative colitis [78 - 81].

These dual effects of the immune system on developing tumors required the reformulation of the immunosurveillance hypothesis, and at 2002 the new term *'cancer immunoediting'* was suggested by Dunn *et al* [14]. According to them, the immune response to cancer development occurs in three phases collectively denoted as the *'three Es'* of cancer immunoediting: elimination (cancer immunos-urveillance), equilibrium (tumor cell variant that has survived the elimination phase are contained, but not fully extinguish), and escape (tumor cell variants selected in the equilibrium phase now can grow in an immunologically integral environment) [82].

CANCER IMMUNOTHERAPY

Immunotherapy is defined as a form of biological therapy that can either activate or inhibit the immune system, assisting the body to eradicate cancer and other disease [83]. In cancer, specifically, the aim of the immunotherapy is to help the body to recognize the cancer cells, activate the immune cells, and break its immune tolerance. The immunotherapy can be classified as active, which aims to activate the adaptive immune system of the patients to destroy tumors and prevent their recurrence; or as adoptive that consists in transferred tumor reactive T cells to the patient and enhances pre-existing immune response [84]. They can also be categorized as nonspecific, which stimulate the host immunity with definite cytokines, DC-based vaccines, NK or NKT cells, or specific mechanisms that use antibodies, γδ T cells, or adoptive αβ T cell therapies [85].

The first adoptive immunotherapy against cancer was tested in 1956 by Dr E Donnall Thomas, who applied a lethal radiation dose in a leukaemia patient followed by bone marrow transplantation (BMT) from the patient's identical twin. The result was the complete disease regression of the disease, stating the principles of the BMT using non-related donor. These principles are still being practiced today as the only curative option for several types of leukaemia.

In 2002, tumor infiltrating lymphocytes (TIL), isolated from a tumor excision, were clinically tested for the first time in a patient with a metastatic melanoma [86]. Four years later, a group had performed a clinical trial using peripheral blood T cells transfected with MART-1 TCR alpha and beta chain gene as TAA. They demonstrated that T cells, which were transduced *ex vivo* with anti-TAA–TCR genes and re-infused in cancer patients, can persist and express the transgene for a prolonged time *in vivo* and mediate the durable regression of large established tumors, becoming a potential method to use in patients for whom TILs are not available [87].

In GI cancers, immunotherapy seems to be a forward step in the path of treatment, and all the diverse strategies are vastly being explored such as 1) stimulation of immunity with inflammatory cytokines, or blocking inhibitory specific check points (*e.g.* CTLA-4 and PD-1) with monoclonal antibodies; 2) vaccines that use tumor antigens, irradiated autologous tumor cells or autologous DCs; 3) adoptive cell therapy with isolated tumor infiltrating lymphocytes [13].

Although preclinical models had demonstrated important results on immunotherapy strategies mainly when associated with other targeted therapeutics, there is a lot of limitations in currently available immunotherapy for GI malignancies, especially the complex interplay between the tumor, the supporting tumor microenvironment, and the immune system (local and systemic). Moreover, it can cause some harmful autoimmune side effects, coming from the damage of peripheral tolerance to antigens expressed by normal tissues. Besides that, GI cancer studies focused on immunotherapy have shown that it can take more than 3 months to observe a radiographic effect in some patients [88].

The success of this approach depends not only on the ability to optimally select cells or genetically modify the same with targeted antigen, but also to induce these cells to proliferate, preserving their effector function and engraftment and homing abilities, and finally does not culminate in collateral effects to the patient. That is probably the reason, despite more than 60 years of research, only in 2010 FDA-approved the first adoptive T-cell therapy protocols for cancer [89].

THERAPY WITH CYTOTOXIC T LYMPHOCYTES

One of the first described adoptive immunotherapy was the infusion of *in vitro* cultured CTL in a melanoma patient [90, 91]. Despite the notable ability of CTL to *in vitro* kill tumor cells, establishment of successful CTL-based therapies is full of obstacles. For instance, some tumor cell variants can less or drastically decrease antigen expression, rising as resistant targets, or the levels of MHC-I molecules can be downregulated on tumor cell surface allowing the escape of MHC-restricted recognition [92]. Although previous results demonstrated that the CTL transfer in cancer patients might have a vaccine-like effect by generating new clones with high anti-tumor response [93], other studies concluded that it is a controversial approach since some of the transferred CTL cells could emerge from an antigen escape variant [94].

It becomes clear that HLA class I expression on the surface of cancer cells, that a requirement for a successful T-cell response since alteration in such expression can affect not only T cell-mediated immunity, but also NK cell activity, culminating in tumorigenic phenotype, metastatic capacity, and so resistance to immunotherapy of various cancer types [95]. A combined therapy with CTL cells and oncolytic adenovirus expressing IL-15 demonstrated an intense antitumor effect on CRC patients. Interleukin-15 was used to activate NK cells and CTL, both able to the lysis tumor target cells [96]. Another option for CTL-based therapy is engineered T cells, to improve anti-tumor effects, and it could be made by chimeric antigen receptors (CAR-T), that will be discussed further.

ADOPTIVE TRANSFER OF TUMOR-INFILTRATING LYMPHOCYTES

Adoptive therapy uses autologous tumor-infiltrating lymphocytes (TILs) isolated from a resected tumor, expanded *in vitro,* and then re-infused back into the patient, to enhance antitumor immunity [97] (Fig. **3A**). This allows manipulation of the T cells by priming them with tumor associated antigens (TAAs) or by transfecting them with recombinant DNA, encoding TCRs specific for definite tumor antigens. TILs can be represented by NK cells, B cells, and various subtypes of T cells (Th1, Th2, Th17, Th9, Treg and CTL), but the best results in many kinds of tumors are associated with accumulation of CD8$^+$ and Th1 cells. At least, in CRC patients, the subtypes and the quantity of TILs are closely associated with the tumor size and with the intensity of inflammatory infiltrates. It was recently demonstrated that there is a decreased number of cells within the inflammatory infiltration in subjects with more advanced disease [98, 99].

It was observed by Halama *et al* [100] that there is a variability of lymphocyte infiltration in the invasive borders of liver metastasis of colorectal cancer. Based on it, they developed a scoring system (density score) in order to predict the patient responsiveness to therapy. According to this group, patients which invasion borders are infiltrated by high numbers of $CD3^+$ cells, associated with a high frequency of $CD8^+$ or granzyme B, are predicted to show a good therapeutic response (grade 4). In opposition, those patients grading 0-2, which presented low density of infiltrating cells in the borders, are predicted to be non-responders to chemotherapy. In addition, the authors stated that evaluation of $CD8^+$ and granzyme B allows a more reliable classification system to predict therapeutic success [101].

Specific Th1 cells are able to respond to gastric cancer antigens and generate cells with the potential to kill cancer cells following re-infusion in patients [102]. Besides, infiltration of $CD3^+$ T cells in GI cancer patients was associated with a higher rate of progression free survival [103]. Pancreatic adenocarcinomas infiltrated with both $CD4^+$ and $CD8^+$ T cells show improved prognosis and significantly increased 5-year survival rate [104]. Hall *et al* successfully isolated and expanded TILs from resected pancreatic adenocarcinomas and observed that under IL-2 stimulation, they present phenotypical markers of previous antigenic experience, including CD69 and CD45RO [105]. Success was also observed in patients with bile duct cancer under chemotherapeutic treatment, adoptively transferred with TILs sensitized with ERBB2-interacting protein [106].

Another attractive strategy for TIL-based cancer therapy is targeting tumor specific mutations, which are biologically important for tumor progression. For example, it was reported that transference of KRAS (KRAS-G12D) mutated T cells obtained from a patient with metastatic colorectal cancer is able to induce the regression of metastatic colon cancer followed by immune evasion [107]. The KRAS oncogene mutation is a recurrent "hot-spot" driver mutation in CRC patients and is also associated with the genesis and progression of many other human cancers [108].

However, these treatments are not immediate therapeutic approach, requiring about six weeks to obtain the quantity and quality of tumor-specific T cells able to destroy tumor cells. T cells must be ready for infusion, making it a methodically difficult approach for large clinical trials until now, except for the melanoma patients [109]. Besides, it is important to consider genomic changes of the tumor, that could, for instance increase the tumor immunogenicity and the immune infiltration as demonstrated in CRC [110].

Side effects were observed in melanoma patients that received T cell infusions, such as vitiligo development of and destruction of melanocytes in the eye and inner ear. It occurs because this therapy consists in the infusion of a large number of high avidity T cells that can also recognize non-tumor associated antigens [111]. In CRC patients, for example, genetically modified T cells with affinity-enhanced TCR to carcinoembryonic antigen (CEA) induced severe colitis in patients since they are also expressed by intestinal epithelial cells [112].

CHIMERIC ANTIGEN-RECEPTOR (CAR)-T CELL THERAPY

Tumor-infiltrating lymphocytes with specific receptors can only be generated from some cancer patients. Then, adoptive T-cell therapy has been amplified and improved by introducing antigen receptors into circulating lymphocytes using retroviral or lentiviral vectors (Fig. **3B**). This can be made by using genes enc-oding T-cell receptors isolated from high avidity tumor-specific T cells called chimeric antigen receptors. Then, T cells are transduced with an artificial receptor gene that contains the antigen-binding region of an antibody, fused with the signal-transduction domains of CD3ζ and co-stimulatory molecules such as CD28 [113]. These cells are expanded *in vitro* T and then, infused into the tumor tissue to attack target cells in an MHC-unrestricted way (Fig. **3B**).

Studies on CAR-T cells' therapy in GI cancer are few. For instance, the thera-peutic efficacy of CAR-T cell therapy in small and large intestine was demons-trated in a CRC murine model of, with no immune-mediated tissue damage. In this study, T cells were transduced with a plasmid expressing guanylyl cyclase C (GUCY2C), a membrane-bounded cyclase gene, whose cell-surface expression is restricted to the apical surfaces of intestinal epithelial cells, being overexpressed in primary and metastatic human CRC [114]. It was also demonstrated that tumor xenografts in mice are completely eliminated after the treatment with CAR-T cells against Her2/neu, a member of the human epidermal growth factor receptor family that mediates normal cell growth and development. CAR-T for CD24, a small heavily glycosylated mucin-like cell surface protein expressed in various malignancies, was also shown to be effective against pancreas cancer cells [115].

T cells carrying two complementary CARs are being investigated since they apparently reduce the risk of collateral toxicity, caused by the recognition of tumor-associated antigens frequently expressed in normal tissues [116]. For example, it was reported that a patient with colon cancer metastasis in the lungs and liver developed lethal pneumonitis after administration of CAR-T cells expressing the tumor antigen ERBB2 (Her-2). It probably occurred because healthy lung cells also express Her-2 gene [117]. Alternatively, it was used as a bispecific antibody (BiAb) which in a specific way, allows the concomitant reaction with a tumor-associated antigen and with a T cell, physically approaching these cells [118].

γδT CELLS BASED IMMUNOTHERAPY

The γδT cell population exhibits peculiar distribution and functions, and plays a significant role in innate immunity against pathogens and tumors. They are also able to crosstalk with DC, and so induce their maturation, functional activation, migration and antigen presentation [119, 120]. The γδT cells also produce high levels of CCR7 for homing to the lymph nodes, where they can activate DC. Active γδT cells have a strong cytotoxic effector activity, produce TNF-α and IFN-γ, and recognize ligands that are not detected by αβT cells, providing an additional pathway to fight the cancer cells [121]. These cells can be isolated from various types of cancer such as CRC, breast, prostate, ovarian and renal carcinomas, and are able to recognize and kill autologous and other related tumors cells, but they do not kill non-transformed cells.

Based on this, γδT cells became an interesting possibility for therapeutic applications. One of the strategies to apply the antitumor activity of γδT cells in cancer immunotherapy is based on the adoptive transference of *ex vivo* expanded γδT cells [122]. These cells can also be stimulated by a concomitant administration of compounds, such as phosphoantigens or aminobisphoshphonates associated with low dose IL-2 [123, 124] (Fig. **3C**).

Classical T-cell based therapy is hindered in GI cancers by the difficulty to identify appropriate target antigens restricted to the tumor cells. Then, γδT cells with their unique features concerned with recognition of conserved non-peptide antigens by an MHC-independent way, open new expectations. Besides, these cells are quickly activated upon antigen exposure, because they are in a pre-activated status, and do not require a previous antigen exposure, as happens with TILs approaches. Moreover, γδT cells are capable to kill colon cancer stem cells (CSCs) pretreated with 5-FU and DXR through mechanisms involving TRAIL /DR5 and NKG2D/MICA/B or ULBPs interactions. Also, the gastric cancer seems to be responsive to γδT cell based therapy [125].

The clinical results showed that patients seem to suffer an exhaustion of γδT cells and immunotherapy based on these cells requirement of *in vitro* reactivation. Oberg et al observed that bispecific antibodies can selectively recruit γδT cells to react against tumor antigens expressed by pancreatic cancer [126], thus optimizing cell reactivity and reducing the requirement of repetitive transference of these cells.

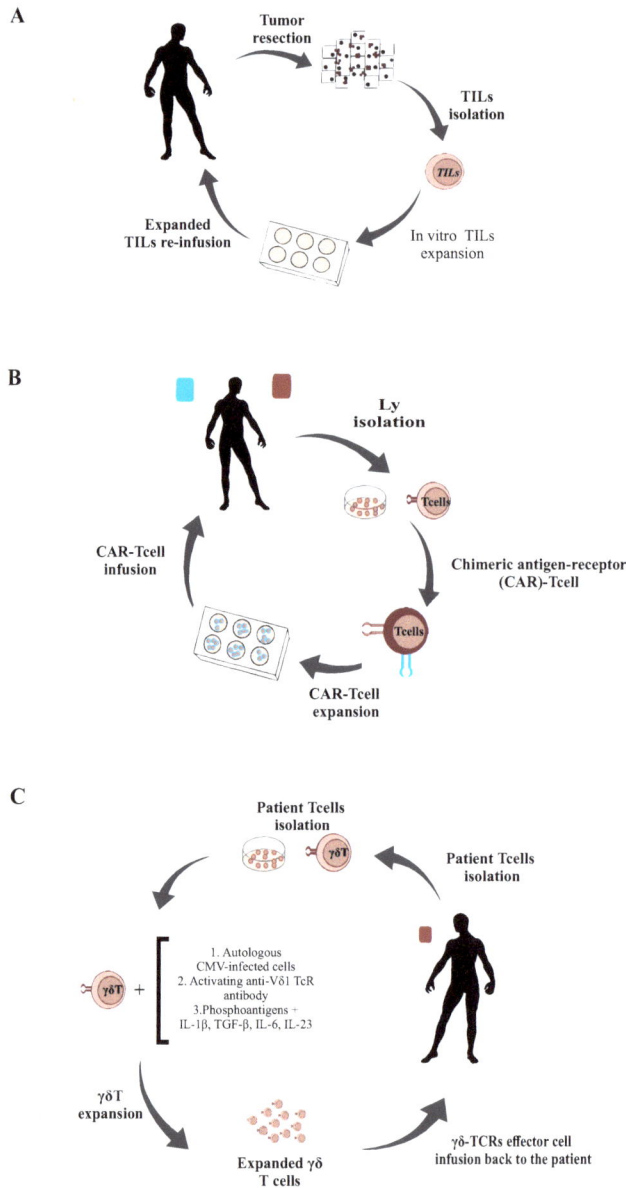

Fig. (3). Three different T cell based approaches of cancer immunotherapy. A) Adoptive transfer of tumor-infiltrating lymphocytes, which consists in enhancing the anti-tumor immunity of a patient reinfusing autologous endogenous tumor-infiltrating lymphocytes that were taken from the resected tumor and expanded *in vitro*. B) The chimeric antigen-receptor (CAR)-T cell therapy transduces an artificial receptor gene to induce *in vitro* expanded T cells to attack tumors in an MHC-unrestricted manner. C) In the γδT cells based immunotherapy, γδT lymphocytes are isolated and *in vitro* expanded and then reinfused to the patient. This expansion could be made by using autologous CMV-infected cells, anti-Vd1 TcR antibody, or using phosphoantigens in the presence of cytokines.

DENDRITIC CELL-BASED VACCINATION

Dendritic cells (DCs) are a heterogeneous population with powerful antigen-presenting cells ability which is derived from bone marrow precursors and work as a link between the peripheral tissue and lymphoid organs. They are the main professional antigen presenting cells due to their unique ability to prime naïve T cells, inducing the clonal expansion of effector cells [127, 128]. There are two different DC categories: plasmacytoid and 'myeloid' DC [129]. The plasmacytoid subset is composed of circulating cells with a lymphoid shape and upon activation by microbial stimuli, they are able to produce large amount of type I interferons, and also activate naïve T cells against exogenous or alloantigens [130 - 132].

Myeloid DC (also referred as conventional DC) derive from CD34$^+$ precursor cells or monocytes [133], and actively control the peripheral tissues and migrate to draining lymph node to present antigens to T cells. There are lymphoid-tissu--resident DC that capture local antigens and present them to local T cells [134]. Due to the paucity of DC naturally found in peripheral blood and the difficult to isolate these cells from human lymphoid organs, most knowledge on DC immunobiology was obtained through the studies with monocyte-derived cells after their differentiation *in vitro* [135].

Monocyte-derived DCs can be loaded with specific antigens and induce the antigen-specific T-cell immunity enhancing the host immunity, becoming a candidate for the antitumor immunotherapy [136]. Antitumor DC-based vaccination consists in loading these cells with tumor associated antigen that will be processed and presented to naive T cells in the context of MHC class I and II molecules. This DC:T contact induces T cell maturation and activation to work as tumor-specific CTL [137].

DC-based vaccines are usually prepared with mature DC (mDC), since there are controversial data about tolerogenic rather than immunogenic role of vaccines prepared with immature DC [138 - 141]. DC maturation can be induced *in vitro* by loading them with a single antigen [142, 143], or by the association of two [144] or more antigens [145]. Among different strategies to deliver antigens to DC, they can be pulsed with proteins [146] or with synthetic peptides representing tumor epitopes [147]. Sensitization with nucleic acids can be made by delivery of TAAs, naked DNA or recombinant viruses (retroviral, adenoviral or vaccinia vectors), or by DC transfection with tumor RNA or synthetic mRNA [85].

Since helper and cytotoxic T cells are induced by antigens presented by MHC-II and MHC-I respectively, targeting these both types of lymphocytes would be required for the induction of a strong and sustained anti-tumor T cell response. However, most clinical DC vaccination studies use synthetic MHC-I-binding peptides [148], mainly to achieve a specific immunization to relevant tumor-epi--opes, and to avoid autoimmune reactivity.

Transfection with synthetic or tumor-derived RNA has been extensively invest-igated, and seems to have several benefits, such as the presentation of MHC class I and sometimes also MHC class II epitopes [149, 150]. RNA delivery seems to be the most potent way to stimulate DC to induce antigen-specific CTLs [151] and it can be done by different techniques, including passive pulsing [152], tran-sferrin receptor-mediated endocytosis, lipofection [153], nucleofection [154] and electroporation [155]. Re-infusion of *ex vivo* generated DCs can be done by intradermal, subcutaneous, intravenous [156], or intranodal injections [157], how-ever, there is no definitive consensus on the best approach to it [158].

There are a restricted number of clinical trials using DC-based vaccines in GI patients despite the good results they demonstrate. This discrepancy probably occurs for the various limitations of this technique, such as the short lifespan of DCs [159], and the fact that the success is mainly restricted by the suppressive tumor micro-environment, that enforces DCs to keep in an immature/tolerogenic state, thereby avoiding T-cell activation [160]. To overcome immune tolerance for successful DC vaccination against GI tract cancers, some authors suggested to load DCs with an altered tumor specific peptide along with appropriate ligand [161], while others have been studying the benefits of the combination of chemo-therapy with immunotherapy [143, 162, 163].

HANDLING REGULATORY T CELLS

Tolerance to self is the biggest obstacle of cancer immunotherapy successes. Central tolerance is stabilized by positive and negative selection of immature lymphocytes in primary lymphoid organs, determining clonal deletion or inac-tivation of self-reactive lymphocytes. Peripheral tolerance, in turn, concerns to mature lymphocytes that are passed by negative selection and left thymus to the periphery. This kind of tolerance is mainly determined and sustained by Treg cells, that functionally suppress other immunocompetent cells [164] and TGFβ, as well as immunosuppressive metabolites such as adenosine.

High peritumoral number of Tregs is associated with advanced-stage tumors and poor overall survival [165]. Besides, *in vitro* Treg depletion from peripheral blood of patients with CRC induces $CD4^+$ and $CD8^+$ T cell responses against TAAs [166]. Clinical approaches to inhibit Tregs include blockade of immune checking points [167], depletion of $CD25^+$ T cells [168] and chemotherapy with low doses of cyclophosphamide [169].

Currently there are three antibodies approved by FDA (US Food and Drug Administration) for clinical use to inhibit the immune checkpoints: Ipilimumab, an anti-CTLA-4 mAb, Nivolumab and Pembrolizumab, both reactive with PD-1. Patients with increased expression of neoantigens concomitantly with accumulation of frame shift or point mutations are more susceptible to the immune checkpoint blockade than patients with mismatch repair-deficient colorectal cancers [170]. Patients who show a pre-existing antitumor immunity before being treated with anti-PD-L1 and anti CTLA4 demonstrate more efficient response to these antibodies [171, 172]. Moreover, in cases of GI cancer in which T cells are not naturally induced, it was demonstrated that immune checkpoint inhibitors are more efficient when combined with some other T cell inducing agents, such as vaccines, as demonstrated with the use of GVAX associated with ipilimumab in the treatment of pancreatic patients [173].

These drugs are only approved for clinical use against metastatic melanoma, while their applications in other cancers, such as CRC, pancreatic and liver cancers are still being investigated. In fact, blocking immune checkpoints protocols failed in GI of cancers, mainly because these cancers weakly induce T cell responses. Specifically, in pancreatic cancer, tumor stroma apparently provides a barrier to infiltration of effector T cells, and when it happens, there is an upregulation of PD-1/PD-L1 pathway, generating an adaptive resistance [87].

GUT MICROBIOME FOR IMMUNOTHERAPY

The intestinal microbiome has been considered as a virtual organ composed by microorganisms exhibiting complex bidirectional crosstalk with the environment and other organ systems [174, 175]. Its composition widely varies between individuals, and plays an important role in the systemic immune development and function [176]. Gut microbiome is a natural, defensive barrier to infection involved in several physiological functions, and plays a large role in maintaining gut homeostasis [177]. In healthy individuals, the intestinal microbiome, mucosal barrier, and immune system are in homeostasis, but when genetic and/or environmental factors cause dysbiosis, there is a disruption of barrier function (leaky gut), leading to inflammation that enhances carcinogenesis (as reviewed by Vindigni *et al*.) [178].

Although the immune checkpoints therapies are already approved by FDA and demonstrate relevant efficacy, an expressive fraction of patients does not respond to these drugs. Investigating the possible reasons for this fall, two groups demonstrated that gut commensals are closely associated with the efficacy of chemotherapies [179, 180], as well as with CTLA-4 and anti-PD-L1 therapies [181, 182]. Anti-CTLA-4 therapy triggers increased apoptosis and proliferation of intestinal epithelial cells that could influence the local microbiota. Both groups demonstrated that gut microbiota can influence the outcome of tumor immunotherapy, and it seems to be related to increased DC activation for starting antitumor T cell responses. This relationship between immune antitumor response and patient's microbiota is a new horizon for the development of immunotherapy adjuvants from bacteria-derived compounds.

CONCLUSION

Immunotherapies using T cells were considered a utopia for a long time, but over the past decade, significant progress has been made in the development of new immunotherapeutic agents such as checkpoint inhibitors and vaccines. These new approaches are gradually being incorporated in the treatment of different cancer types. Advances in the knowledge about T cell functions, activation pathways and their role in the battle against cancer renew the hope of medical and scientific community, and patients, but there is a long road to achieve the cancer cure. Researchers all around the world are looking for answers to critical questions *"why these therapies are more effective for some patients than to others?"* and *"why these therapies work best for a specific type of cancer and not for others.* Therefore, efficacy of cancer immunotherapy depends on a deeper understanding of the relationship between the immune system and tumor microenvironment.

CONFLICT OF INTEREST

The authors declare no conflict of interest, financial or otherwise.

ACKNOWLEDGEMENTS

The study was supported by a grant from the regional contribution of "The Programma Attuativo Regionale (Toscana) funded by FAS (now FSC), the Italian Ministry of University and Research (MIUR) and the Foundation 'Ente Cassa di Risparmio di Firenze'.

REFERENCES

[1]   Siegel RL, Miller KD, Jemal A. Cancer statistics, 2016. CA Cancer J Clin 2016; 66(1): 7-30.

[2]   Global Burden of Disease Cancer Collaboration. Global, Regional, and National Cancer Incidence, Mortality, Years of Life Lost, Years Lived With Disability, and Disability-Adjusted Life-years for 32 Cancer Groups, 1990 to 2015: A Systematic Analysis for the Global Burden of Disease Study. JAMA Oncol 2016.

[3]   Yi M, Xu J, Liu P, Chang GJ, Du XL, Hu CY, *et al.* Comparative analysis of lifestyle factors, screening test use, and clinicopathologic features in association with survival among Asian Americans with colorectal cancer. Br J Cancer 2013; 108(7): 1508-14.

[4]   Fang X, Wei J, He X, An P, Wang H, Jiang L, *et al.* Landscape of dietary factors associated with risk of gastric cancer: A systematic review and dose-response meta-analysis of prospective cohort studies.

Eur J Cancer 51(18): 2820-32.

[5]   American Cancer Society. Cancer Facts & Figures 2016. Atlanta: American Cancer Society 2016.

[6]   Duarte-Salles T, Fedirko V, Stepien M, Aleksandrova K, Bamia C, Lagiou P, *et al.* Dietary fat, fat subtypes and hepatocellular carcinoma in a large European cohort. Int J Cancer 2015; 137: 2715-28.

[7]   Hoppes WL, Lerner PI. Nonenterococcal group-D streptococcal endocarditis caused by Streptococcus bovis. Ann Intern Med 1974; 81: 588-93.

[8]   Handa O, Naito Y, Yoshikawa T. Helicobacter pylori: a ROSinducing bacterial species in the stomach. Inflamm Res 2010; 59: 997-1003.

[9]   Kanwal F, Kramer JR, Ilyas J, Duan Z, El-Serag HB. HCV genotype 3 is associated with an increased risk of cirrhosis and hepatocellular cancer in a national sample of US Veterans with HCV. Hepatology 2014; 60: 98-105.

[10]   Kidane D, Chae WJ, Czochor J, *et al.* Interplay between DNA repair and inflammation, and the link to câncer. Crit Rev Biochem Mol Biol 2014; 49(2): 116-39.

[11]   D'Angelica M, Gonen M, Brennan MF, Turnbull AD, Bains M, Karpeh MS. Patterns of initial recurrence in completely resected gastric adenocarcinoma. Ann Surg 2004; 240: 808-16.

[12]   Macdonald JS, Smalley SR, Benedetti J, Hundahl SA, Estes NC, Stemmermann GN, *et al.* Chemoradiotherapy after Surgery Compared with Surgery Alone for adenocarcinoma of the Stomach or Gastroesophageal Junction. N Engl J Med 2001; 345: 725-30.

[13]   Pernot S, Terme M, Voron T, *et al.* Colorectal cancer and immunity: What we know and perspectives. World J Gastroenterol 2014; 20(14): 3738-50.

[14]   Dunn GP, Bruce AT, Ikeda H, Old LJ, Schreiber RD. Cancer immunoediting: from immunosurveillance to tumor escape. Nat Immunol 2002; 3(11): 991-8.

[15]   Boon T, Cerottini JC, Van denEynde B, van der Bruggen P, Van Pel A. Tumor antigensrecognizedby T lymphocytes. Annu Rev Immunol 1994; 12: 337-65.

[16]   Matsushita H, Vesely MD, Koboldt DC, Rickert CG, Uppaluri R, Magrini VJ, *et al.* Cancer exome analysis reveals a T-cell-dependent mechanism of cancer immunoediting. Nature 2012; 482: 400-4.

[17]   Lennerz V, Fatho M, Gentilini C, Frye RA, Lifke A, Ferel D, *et al.* The response of autologous T cells to a human melanoma is dominated by mutated neoantigens. Proc Natl Acad Sci USA 2005; 102: 16013-8.

[18]   Galon J, Costes A, Sanchez-Cabo F, Kirilovsky A, Mlecnik B, Lagorce-Pagès C, *et al.* Type, density, and location of immune cells within human colorectal tumors predict clinical outcome. Science 2006; 313(5795): 1960-4.

[19]   Alberts B, Johnson A, Lewis J, Raff M, Roberts K, Walter P. Molecular biology of the cell. 4th ed., New York: Garland Science 2002.

[20]   Inston N, Drayson M, Ready A, Cockwell P. Serial changes in the expression of CXCR3 and CCR5 on peripheral blood lymphocytes following human renal transplantation. Exp Clin Transplant 2007; 5(2): 638-42.

[21]   Zou W. Immunosuppressive networks in the tumor environment and their therapeutic relevance. Nat Rev Cancer 2005; 5: 263-74.

[22]   Ekkens MJ, Shedlock DJ, Jung E, Troy A, Pearce EL, Shen H, *et al.* Th1 and Th2 cells help CD8 T-cell responses. Infect Immun 2007; 75(5): 2291-6.

[23]   Robinson DS, Hamid Q, Ying S, Tsicopoulos A, Barkans J, Bentley AM, *et al.* Predominant TH2-like bronchoalveolar T-lymphocyte population in atopic asthma. N Engl J Med 1992; 326(5): 298-304.

[24]   Atarashi K, Tanoue T, Ando M, Kamada N, Nagano Y, Narushima S, *et al.* Th17 Cell Induction by Adhesion of Microbes to Intestinal Epithelial Cells. Cell 2015; 163(2): 367-80.

[25]   Leipe J, Grunke M, Dechant C, Reindl C, Kerzendorf U, Schulze-Koops H, *et al.* Role of Th17 cells in human autoimmune arthritis. Arthritis Rheum 2010; 62(10): 2876-85.

[26]   Slebioda TJ, Bojarska-Junak A, Stanisławowski M, Cyman M, Wierzbicki PM, Roliński J, *et al.* TL1A as a potential local inducer of IL17A expression in colon mucosa of inflammatory bowel disease patients. Scand J Immunol 2015; 82(4): 352-60.

[27]   Ulrich CM1. Bigler J, Potter JD. Non-steroidal anti-inflammatory drugs for cancer prevention: promise, perils and pharmacogenetics. Nat Rev Cancer 2006; 6(2): 130-40.

[28]   Numasaki M, Fukushi J, Ono M, Narula SK, Zavodny PJ, Kudo T, *et al.* Interleukin-17 promotes angiogenesis and tumor growth. Blood 2003; 101: 2620-7.

[29]   Chtanova T, Tangye SG, Newton R, Frank N, Hodge MR, Rolph MS, *et al.* T follicular helper cells express a distinctive transcriptional profile, reflecting their role as non-Th1/Th2 effector cells that provide help for B cells. J Immunol 2004; 173(1): 68-78.

[30]   Crotty S. Follicular helper CD4 T cells (TFH). Annu Rev Immunol 2011; 29: 621-63.

[31]   Johansson-Lindbom B, Ingvarsson S, Borrebaeck CA. Germinal centers regulate human Th2 development. J Immunol 2003; 171(4): 1657-66.

[32]   Veldhoen M, Uyttenhove C, van Snick J, Helmby H, Westendorf A, Buer J, *et al.* Transforming growth factor-beta 'reprograms' the differentiation of T helper 2 cells and promotes an interleukin 9-producing subset. Nat Immunol 2008; 9(12): 1341-6.

[33]   Anuradha R1. IL-4-, TGF-β-, and IL-1-dependent expansion of parasite antigen-specific Th9 cells is associated with clinical pathology in human lymphatic filariasis. J Immunol 2013; 191(5): 2466-73.

[34]   Xie J, Lotoski LC, Choonieedass R, Su RC, Simons FE, Liem J, *et al.* Elevated antigen-driven IL-9 responses are prominent in peanut allergic humans. PLoS One 2012; 7(10): e45377.

[35]   Sakaguchi S, Sakaguchi N, Asano M, Itoh M, Toda M. Immunologic self-tolerance maintained by activated T cells expressing IL-2 receptor α-chains (CD25): breakdown of a single mechanism of self-tolerance causes various autoimmune diseases. J Immunol 1995; 155: 1151.

[36]   Thornton AM, Shevach EM. CD4 CD25 immunoregulatory T cells suppress polyclonal T cell activation *in vitro* by inhibiting interleukin 2 production. J Exp Med 1998; 188: 287.

[37]   Rudensky AY. Regulatory T cells and Foxp3. Immunol Rev 2011; 241(1): 260-8.

[38]   Restifo NP, Dudley ME, Rosenberg AS. Adoptive immunotherapy for cancer: harnessing the T cell response. Nat Rev Immunol 2012; 12: 269-81.

[39]   Jones J, Morgan BP. Killing of cells by perforin. Resistance to killing is not due to diminished binding of perforin to the cell membrane. Biochem J 1991; 280(Pt 1): 199-204.

[40]   Henkart PA. Mechanism of lymphocyte-mediated cytotoxicity. Annu Rev Immunol 1985; 3: 31-58.

[41]   Grossman WJ, Revell PA, Lu ZW, Johnson H, Bredemeyer AJ, Ley TJ. The orphan granzymes of humans and mice. Curr Opin Immunol 2003; 15: 544-52.

[42]   Chowdhury D, Lieberman J. Death by a thousand cuts: granzyme pathways of programmed cell death. Annu Rev Immunol 2008; 26: 389-420.

[43]   Carlsson B, Forsberg O, Bengtsson M, Tötterman TH, Essand M. Characterization of human prostate and breast cancer cell lines for experimental T cell-based immunotherapy. Prostate 2007; 67(4): 389-95.

[44]   Hung K, Hayashi R, Lafond-Walker A, Lowenstein C, Pardoll D, Levitsky H. The central role of CD4(+) T cells in the antitumorimmune response. J Exp Med 1998; 188: 2357-68.

[45]   Goedert JJ. The epidemiology of acquired immunodeficiency syndrome malignancies. Semin Oncol 2000; 27(4): 390-401.

[46]   Kaneno R. Role of natural killer cells in antitumor resistance. ARBS Annu Rev Biomed Sci 2005; 7: 127-48.

[47]   Timonen T, Saksela E, Ranki A, Häyry P. Fractionation, morphological and functional characterization of effector cells responsible for human natural killer activity against cell-line targets. Cell Immunol 1979; 48(1): 133-48.

[48]   Lotzová E, Ades EW. Natural killer cells: definition, heterogeneity, lytic mechanism, functions and clinical application. Highlights of the Fifth International Workshop on natural killer cells, Hilton Head Island, N.C., March 1988. Nat Immun Cell Growth Regul 1989; 8(1): 1-9.

[49]   Kobayashi M, Fitz L, Ryan M, Hewick RM, Clark SC, Chan S, *et al.* Identification and purification of natural killer cell stimulatory factor (NKSF), a cytokine with multiple biologic effects on human lymphocytes. J Exp Med 1989; 170(3): 827-45.

[50]   Timonen T, Saksela E. Isolation of human NK cells by density gradient centrifugation. J Immunol Methods 1980; 36(3-4): 285-91.

[51]   Sutlu T, Alici E. Natural killer cell-based immunotherapy in cancer: current insights and future prospects. J Intern Med 2009; 266(2): 154-81.

[52]   Di Santo JP. Functionally distinct NK-cell subsets: developmental origins and biological implications. Eur J Immunol 2008; 38: 2948-51.

[53]   Wu J, Lanier LL. Natural killer cells and cancer. Adv Cancer Res 2003; 90: 127-56.

[54]   Baker GJ, Chockley P, Yadav VN, Doherty R, Ritt M, Sivaramakrishnan S, *et al.* Natural killer cells eradicate galectin-1-deficient glioma in the absence of adaptive immunity. Cancer Res 2014; 74: 5079-90.

[55]   Trinchieri G. Biology of natural killer cells. Adv Immunol 1989; 47: 187-376.

[56]   Cooper MA, Fehniger TA, Caligiuri MA. The biology of human natural killer-cell subsets. Trends Immunol 2001; 22(11): 633-40.

[57]   Natarajan K, Dimasi N, Wang J, Mariuzza RA, Margulies DH. Structure and function of natural killer cell receptors: multiple molecular solutions to self, nonself discrimination. Annu Rev Immunol 2002; 20: 853-85.

[58]   Wu J, Song Y, Bakker AB, Bauer S, Spies T, Lanier LL, *et al.* An activating immunoreceptor complex formed by NKG2D and DAP10. Science 1999; 285(5428): 730-2.

[59]   Menier C, Riteau B, Carosella ED, Rouas-Freiss N. MICA triggering signal for NK cell tumor lysis is counteracted by HLA-G1-mediated inhibitory signal. Int J Cancer 2002; 100(1): 63-70.

[60]   Bauer S, Groh V, Wu J, Steinle A, Phillips JH, Lanier LL, *et al.* Activation of NK cells and T cells by NKG2D, a receptor for stress-inducible MICA. Science 1999; 285(5428): 727-9.

[61]   Rincon-Orozco B, Kunzmann V, Wrobel P, Kabelitz D, Steinle A, Herrmann T. Activation of V gamma 9V delta 2 T cells by NKG2D. J Immunol 2005; 175(4): 2144-51.

[62]   Horny HP, Horst HA. Lymphoreticular infiltrates in adenocarcinoma of the large intestine. Pathol Res Pract 1987; 182(2): 222-7.

[63]   Adachi W, Usuda N, Sugenoya A, Iida F. Immune-competent cells of regional lymph nodes in colorectal cancer patients: II. Immunohistochemical analysis of Leu-7+ cells. J Surg Oncol 1990; 45(4): 234-41.

[64]   Coca S, Perez-Piqueras J, Martinez D, Colmenarejo A, Saez MA, Vallejo C, *et al.* The prognostic significance of intratumoral natural killer cells in patients with colorectal carcinoma. Cancer 1997; 79(12): 2320-8.

[65] Ishigami S, Natsugoe S, Tokuda K, Nakajo A, Xiangming C, Iwashige H, *et al.* Clinical impact of intratumoral natural killer cell and dendritic cell infiltration in gastric cancer. Cancer Lett 2000; 159(1): 103-8.

[66] Aparicio-Pagés NM, Verspaget HW, Peña SA, Lamers CB. Impaired local natural killer cell activity in human colorectal carcinomas. Cancer Immunol Immunother 1989; 28(4): 301-4.

[67] Vujanovic NL, Basse P, Herberman RB, Whiteside TL. Antitumor Functions of Natural Killer Cells and Control of Metastases. Methods 1996; 9(2): 394-408.

[68] Cho D, Campana D. Expansion and activation of natural killer cells for cancer immunotherapy. Korean J Lab Med 2009; 29(2): 89-96.

[69] Bendelac A, Savage PB, Teyton L. The biology of NKT cells. Annu Rev Immunol 2007; 25: 297-336.

[70] Taniguchi M, Seino K, Nakayama T. The NKT cell system: bridging innate and acquired immunity. Nat Immunol 2003; 4(12): 1164-5.

[71] Seino K, Motohashi S, Fujisawa T, Nakayama T, Taniguchi M. Natural killer T cell-mediated antitumor immune responses and their clinical applications. Cancer Sci 2006; 97(9): 807-12.

[72] Terabe M, Berzofsky JA. The immunoregulatory role of type I and type II NKT cells in cancer and other diseases. Cancer immunology, immunotherapy. CII 2014; 63(3): 199-213.

[73] Kronenberg M, Gapin L. The unconventional lifestyle of NKT cells. Nat Rev Immunol 2002; 2(8): 557-68.

[74] Salama P, Platell C. Host response to colorectal cancer. ANZ J Surg 2008; 78(9): 745-53.

[75] Wang X, Lin Y. Tumor necrosis factor and cancer, buddies or foes? Acta Pharmacol Sin 2008; 29(11): 1275-88.

[76] Waugh DJ, Wilson C. The interleukin-8 pathway in cancer. Clin Cancer Res 2008; 14(21): 6735-41.

[77] Itakura J, Ishiwata T, Shen B, Kornmann M, Korc M. Concomitant over-expression of vascular endothelial growth factor and its receptors in pancreatic cancer. Int J Cancer 2000; 85: 27-34.

[78] Winther KV, Jess T, Langholz E, Munkholm P, Binder V. Long-term risk of cancer in ulcerative colitis: a population-based cohort study from Copenhagen County. Clin Gastroenterol Hepatol 2004; 2(12): 1088-95.

[79] Farraye FA, Odze RD, Eaden J, Itzkowitz SH. AGA technical review on the diagnosis and management of colorectal neoplasia in inflammatory bowel disease 2010.

[80] Ullman TA, Itzkowitz SH. Intestinal inflammation and cancer. Gastroenterology 2011; 140(6): 1807-16.

[81] Lutgens MW, van Oijen MG, van der Heijden GJ, Vleggaar FP, Siersema PD, Oldenburg B. Declining risk of colorectal cancer in inflammatory bowel disease: an updated meta-analysis of population-based cohort studies. Inflamm Bowel Dis 2013; 19(4): 789-99.

[82] Dunn GP, Old LJ, Schreiber RD. The three Es of cancer immunoediting. Annu Rev Immunol 2004; 22: 329-60.

[83] National Cancer Institute. Immunotherapy: Using the Immune System to Treat Cancer. Available from: https://www.cancer.gov/research/areas/treatment/immunotherapy-using-immune-system [Accessed 25th January 2017].

[84] Farkona S, Diamandis EP, Blasutig IM. Cancer immunotherapy: the beginning of the end of cancer? BMC Med. 201; 14:73.

[85] Amedei A, D'Elios MM. Cancer: Recent development of cell-based immunotherapy. In: Facinelli BC, Ed. Immunotherapy: Activation, suppression and treatments. New York, NY: Nova Biomedical 2010; pp. 77-129.

[86] Dudley ME, Wunderlich JR, Robbins PF, Yang JC, Hwu P, Schwartzentruber DJ, *et al.* Cancer regression and autoimmunity in patients after clonal repopulation with antitumor lymphocytes. Science 2002; 298: 850-4.

[87] Morgan RA, Dudley ME, Wunderlich JR, Hughes MS, Yang JC, Sherry RM, *et al.* Cancer regression in patients after transfer of genetically engineered lymphocytes. Science 2006; 314: 126-9.

[88] Wang J, Reiss KA, Khatri R, Jaffee E, Laheru D. Immune Therapy in GI Malignancies: A Review. J Clin Oncol 2015; 33(16): 1745-53.

[89] Snyder A, Tepper JE, Slovin SF. Perspectives on immunotherapy in prostate cancer and solid tumors: where is the future? Semin Oncol 2013; 40: 347-60.

[90] van der Bruggen P, Traversari C, Chomez P, Lurquin C, De Plaen E, Van den Eynde B, *et al.* A gene encoding an antigen recognized by cytolytic T lymphocytes on a human melanoma. Science 1991; 254(5038): 1643-7.

[91] June CH. Principles of adoptive T cell cancer therapy. J Clin Invest 2007; 117(5): 1204-12.

[92] Garrido F, Ruiz-Cabello F, Aptsiauri N. Rejection *versus* escape: the tumor MHC dilemma. Cancer Immunol Immunother 2017; 66(2): 259-71.

[93] Vignard V, Lemercier B, Lim A, Pandolfino MC, Guilloux Y, Khammari A, *et al.* Adoptive transfer of tumor-reactive Melan-A-specific CTL clones in melanoma patients is followed by increased frequencies of additional Melan-A-specific T cells. J Immunol 2005; 175(7): 4797-805.

[94] Marincola FM, Jaffee EM, Hicklin DJ, Ferrone S. Escape of human solid tumors from T-cell recognition: molecular mechanisms and functional significance. Adv Immunol 2000; 74: 181-273.

[95] Thor Straten P, Garrido F. Targetless T cells in cancer immunotherapy. J Immunother Cancer 2016; 4: 23.

[96] Yan Y, Li S, Jia T, Du X, Xu Y, Zhao Y, *et al.* Combined therapy with CTL cells and oncolytic adenovirus expressing IL-15-induced enhanced antitumor activity. Tumour Biol 2015; 36(6): 4535-43.

[97] Rosenberg SA, Restifo NP. Adoptive cell transfer as personalized immunotherapy for human cancer. Science 2015; 348: 62-8.

[98] Funada Y, Noguchi T, Kikuchi R, Takeno S, Uchida Y, Gabbert HE. Prognostic significance of CD8+ T cell and macrophage peritumoral infiltration in colorectal cancer. Oncol Rep 2003; 10: 309-13.

[99] Łaskowski P, Klim B, Ostrowski K, Szkudlarek M, Litwiejko-Pietryńczak E, Kitlas K, *et al.* Local inflammatory response in colorectal cancer. Pol J Pathol 2016; 67(2): 163-71.

[100] Halama N, Michel S, Kloor M, Zoernig I, Benner A, Spille A, *et al.* Localization and density of immune cells in the invasive margin of human colorectal cancer liver metastases are prognostic for response to chemotherapy. Cancer Res 2011; 71(17): 5670-7.

[101] Halama N, Michel S, Kloor M, Zoernig I, Benner A, Spille A, *et al.* Localization and density of immune cells in the invasive margin of human colorectal cancer liver metastases are prognostic for response to chemotherapy. Cancer Res 2011; 71(17): 5670-7.

[102] Amedei A, Niccolai E, Della Bella C, Cianchi F, Trallori G, Benagiano M, *et al.* Characterization of tumor antigen peptidespecific T cells isolated from the neoplastic tissue of patients with gastric adenocarcinoma. Cancer Immunol Immunother 2009; 58: 1819-30.

[103] Rusakiewicz S, Semeraro M, Sarabi M, Desbois M, Locher C, Mendez R, *et al.* Immune infiltrates are prognostic factors in localized gastrointestinal stromal tumors. Cancer Res 2013; 73(12): 3499-510.

[104] Sideras K, Braat H, Kwekkeboom J, *et al.* Role of the immune system in pancreatic cancer progression and immune modulating treatment strategies. Cancer Treat Rev 2014; 40(4): 513-22.

[105] Hall M, Liu H, Malafa M, *et al.* Expansion of tumor-infiltrating lymphocytes (TIL) from human pancreatic tumors. J Immunother Cancer 2016; 18(4): 61.

[106]   Tran E, Turcotte S, Gros A, Robbins PF, Lu YC, Dudley ME, *et al.* Cancer immunotherapy based on mutation-specific CD4+ T cells in a patient with epithelial cancer. Science 2014; 344(6184): 641-5.

[107]   Tran E, Robbins PF, Lu YC, Prickett TD, Gartner JJ, Jia L, *et al.* T-Cell Transfer Therapy Targeting Mutant KRAS in Cancer. N Engl J Med 2016; 8(375): 2255-62.

[108]   Tie J, Lipton L, Desai J, Gibbs P, Jorissen RN, Christie M, *et al.* KRAS mutation is associated with lung metastasis in patients with curatively resected colorectal cancer. Clin Cancer Res 2011; 17(5): 1122-30.

[109]   Niccolai E, Taddei A, Prisco D, Amedei A. Gastric cancer and the epoch of immunotherapy approaches. World J Gastroenterol 2015; 21(19): 5778-93.

[110]   Giannakis M, Mu XJ, Shukla SA, Qian ZR, Cohen O, Nishihara R, *et al.* Genomic Correlates of Immune-Cell Infiltrates in Colorectal Carcinoma 2016.

[111]   Johnson LA, Morgan RA, Dudley ME, Cassard L, Yang JC, Hughes MS, *et al.* Gene therapy with human and mouse T-cell receptors mediates cancer regression and targets normal tissues expressing cognate antigen. Blood 2009; 114(3): 535-46.

[112]   Parkhurst MR, Yang JC, Langan RC, Dudley ME, Nathan DA, Feldman SA, *et al.* T cells targeting carcinoembryonic antigen can mediate regression of metastatic colorectal cancer but induce severe transient colitis. Mol Ther 2011; 19: 620-6.

[113]   Maus MV, Grupp SA, Porter DL, June CH. Antibody-modified T cells: CARs take the front seat for hematologic malignancies. Blood 2014; 123(17): 2625-35.

[114]   Magee MS, Kraft CL, Abraham TS, Baybutt TR, Marszalowicz GP, Li P, *et al.* GUCY2C-directed CAR-T cells oppose colorectal cancer metastases without autoimmunity. OncoImmunology 2016; 5(10): e1227897.

[115]   Maliar A, Servais C, Waks T, Chmielewski M, Lavy R, Altevogt P, *et al.* Redirected T cells that target pancreatic adenocarcinoma antigens eliminate tumors and metastases in mice. Gastroenterology 2012; 143(5): 1375-84.e1-5.

[116]   Chen C, Li K, Jiang H, Song F, Gao H, Pan X, *et al.* Development of T cells carrying two complementary chimeric antigen receptors against glypican-3 and asialoglycoprotein receptor 1 for the treatment of hepatocellular carcinoma. Cancer Immunol Immunother 2016.

[117]   Morgan RA, Yang JC, Kitano M, Dudley ME, Laurencot CM, Rosenberg SA. Case report of a serious adverse event following the administration of T cells transduced with a chimeric antigen receptor recognizing ERBB2. Mol Ther 2010; 18: 843-51.

[118]   Topp MS, Kufer P, Gökbuget N, Goebeler M, Klinger M, Neumann S, *et al.* Targeted therapy with the T-cell-engaging antibody blinatumomab of chemotherapy-refractory minimal residual disease in B-lineage acute lymphoblastic leukemia patients results in high response rate and prolonged leukemia-free survival. J Clin Oncol 2011; 29(18): 2493-8.

[119]   Girardi M. Immunosurveillance and immunoregulation by gammadelta T cells. J Invest Dermatol 2006; 126(1): 25-31.

[120]   Münz C, Steinman RM, Fujii S. Dendritic cell maturation by innate lymphocytes: coordinated stimulation of innate and adaptive immunity. J Exp Med 2005; 202(2): 203-7.

[121]   Hayday AC. γδT cells: a right time and a right place for a conserved third way of protection. Annu Rev Immunol 2000; 18: 975-1026.

[122]   Silva-Santos B, Serre K, Norell H. γδ T cells in cancer. Nat Rev Immunol 2015; 15(11): 683-91.

[123]   Pfeffer K, Schoel B, Gulle H, Kaufmann SH, Wagner H. Primary responses of human T cells to mycobacteria: a frequent set of gamma/delta T cells are stimulated by proteaseresistant ligands. Eur J Immunol 1990; 20(5): 1175-9.

[124] Corvaisier M, Moreau-Aubry A, Diez E, Bennouna J, Mosnier JF, Scotet E, *et al.* Vg9Vy2T cell response to colon carcinoma cells. J Immunol 2005; 175(8): 5481-8.

[125] Mao C, Mou X, Zhou Y, Yuan G, Xu C, Liu H, *et al.* Tumor-activated TCRγδ⁺ T cells from gastric cancer patients induce the antitumor immune response of TCRαβ⁺ T cells *via* their antigen-presenting cell-like effects. J Immunol Res 2014; 2014: 593562.

[126] Oberg HH, Peipp M, Kellner C, Sebens S, Krause S, Petrick D, *et al.* Novel bispecific antibodies increase γδ T-cell cytotoxicity against pancreatic cancer cells. Cancer Res 2014; 74(5): 1349-60.

[127] Steinman RM. The dendritic cell system and its role in immunogenicity. Annu Rev Immunol 1991; 9: 271-9.

[128] Avigan D. Dendritic cells: development, function and potential use for cancer immunotherapy. Blood Rev 1999; 13(1): 51-64.

[129] Villadangos JA, Schnorrer P. Intrinsic and cooperative antigenpresenting functions of dendritic-cell subsets *in vivo.* Nat Rev Immunol 2007; 7: 543-55.

[130] Soumelis V, Liu YJ. From plasmacytoid to dendritic cell: morphological and functional switches during plasmacytoid pre-dendritic cell differentiation. Eur J Immunol 2006; 36: 2286-92.

[131] Grouard G, Rissoan MC, Filgueira L, Durand I, Banchereau J, Liu YJ. The enigmatic plasmacytoid T cells develop into dendritic cells with interleukin (IL)-3 and CD40-ligand. J Exp Med 1997; 185: 1101-11.

[132] Benitez-Ribas D, Adema GJ, Winkels G, *et al.* Plasmacytoid dendritic cells of melanoma patients present exogenous proteins to CD4+ T cells after Fc gamma RII-mediated uptake. J Exp Med 2006; 203: 1629-35.

[133] Randolph GJ, Beaulieu S, Lebecque S, Steinman RM, Muller WA. Differentiation of monocytes into dendritic cells in a model of transendothelial trafficking. Science 1998; 282: 480-3.

[134] Shortman K, Naik SH. Steady-state and inflammatory dendritic-cell development. Nat Rev Immunol 2007; 7: 19-30.

[135] Banchereau J, Palucka AK, Dhodapkar M, Burkeholder S, Taquet N, Rolland A, *et al.* Immune and clinical responses in patients with metastatic melanoma to CD34(+) progenitor-derived dendritic cell vaccine. Cancer Res 2001; 61: 6451-8.

[136] Jahnisch H, Fussel S, Kiessling A, Wehner R, Zastrow S, Bachmann M, *et al.* Dendritic cell-based immunotherapy for prostate Cancer 2010.

[137] Mescher MF, Curtsinger JM, Agarwal P, Casey KA, Gerner M, Hammerbeck CD, *et al.* Signals required for programming effector and memory development by CD8+ T cells. Immunol Rev 2006; 211: 81-92.

[138] Steinman RM, Nussenzweig MC. Avoiding horror autotoxicus: the importance of dendritic cells in peripheral T cell tolerance. Proc Natl Acad Sci USA 2002; 99: 351-8.

[139] Dhodapkar MV, Steinman RM, Krasovsky J, Munz C, Bhardwaj N. Antigen-specific inhibition of effector T cell function in humans after injection of immature dendritic cells. J Exp Med 2001; 193: 233-8.

[140] Jonuleit H, Giesecke-Tuettenberg A, Tuting T, Thurner-Schuler B, Stuge TB, Paragnik L, *et al.* A comparison of two types of dendritic cell as adjuvants for the induction of melanomaspecific T-cell responses in humans following intranodal injection. Int J Cancer 2001; 93: 243-51.

[141] Mann DL, Celluzzi CM, Hankey KG, Harris KM, Watanabe R, Hasumi K. Combining conventional therapies with intratumoral injection of autologous dendritic cells and activated T cells to treat patients with advanced cancers. Ann N Y Acad Sci 2009; 1174: 41-50.

[142] Morse MA, Nair SK, Mosca PJ, Hobeika AC, Clay TM, Deng Y, *et al.* Immunotherapy with autologous, human dendritic cells transfected with carcinoembryonic antigen mRNA. Cancer Invest

2003; 21(3): 341-9.

[143]   Lesterhuis WJ, De Vries IJ, Schreibelt G, Schuurhuis DH, Aarntzen EH, De Boer A, *et al.* Immunogenicity of dendritic cells pulsed with CEA peptide or transfected with CEA mRNA for vaccination of colorectal cancer patients. Anticancer Res 2010; 30(12): 5091-7.

[144]   Morse MA, Niedzwiecki D, Marshall JL, Garrett C, Chang DZ, Aklilu M, *et al.* A randomized phase II study of immunization with dendritic cells modified with poxvectors encoding CEA and MUC1 compared with the same poxvectors plus GM-CSF for resected metastatic colorectal cancer. Ann Surg 2013; 258(6): 879-86.

[145]   Kavanagh B, Ko A, Venook A, *et al.* Vaccination of metastatic colorectal cancer patients with matured dendritic cells loaded with multiple major histocompatibility complex class I peptides. J Immunother 2007; 30(7): 762-72.

[146]   Kaneno R, Shurin GV, Kaneno FM, Naiditch H, Luo J, Shurin MR. Chemotherapeutic agents in low noncytotoxic concentrations increase immunogenicity of human colon cancer cells. Cell Oncol (Dordr) 2011; 34(2): 97-106.

[147]   Keogh E, Fikes J, Southwood S, Celis E, Chesnut R, Sette A. Identification of new epitopes from four different tumor-associated antigens: recognition of naturally processed epitopes correlates with HLA-A*0201-binding affinity. J Immunol 2001; 167: 787-96.

[148]   Lesterhuis WJ, Aarntzen EH, De Vries IJ, *et al.* Dendritic cell vaccines in melanoma: from promise to proof? Crit Rev Oncol Hematol 2008; 66(2): 118-34.

[149]   Kyte JA, Aamdal S, Dueland S, Sæbøe-Larsen S, Inderberg EM, Madsbu UE, *et al.* Immune response and long-term clinical outcome in advanced melanoma patients vaccinated with tumor-mRN--transfected dendritic cells. OncoImmunology 2016; 5(11): e1232237.

[150]   Tyagi RK, Parmar R, Patel N. A generic RNA pulsed DC based approach for developing therapeutic intervention against Nasopharyngeal Carcinoma 2016.

[151]   Nencioni A, Grünebach F, Schmidt SM, *et al.* The use of dendritic cells in cancer immunotherapy. Crit Rev Oncol Hematol 2008; 65(3): 191-9.

[152]   Boczkowski D, Nair SK, Snyder D, Gilboa E. Dendritic cells pulsed with RNA are potent antigen-presenting cells *in vitro* and *in vivo.* J Exp Med 1996; 184(2): 465-72.

[153]   Grünebach F, Müller MR, Nencioni A, Brossart P. Delivery of tumor-derived RNA for the induction of cytotoxic T-lymphocytes. Gene Ther 2003; 10(5): 367-74.

[154]   Gresch O, Engel FB, Nesic D, Tran TT, England HM, Hickman ES, *et al.* New non-viral method for gene transfer into primary cells. Methods 2004; 33(2): 151-63.

[155]   Javorovic M, Pohla H, Frankenberger B, Wölfel T, Schendel DJ. RNA transfer by electroporation into mature dendritic cells leading to reactivation of effector-memory cytotoxic T lymphocytes: a quantitative analysis. Mol Ther 2005; 12(4): 734-43.

[156]   Curti A, Tosi P, Comoli P, Terragna C, Ferri E, Cellini C, *et al.* Phase I/II clinical trial of sequential subcutaneous and intravenous delivery of dendritic cell vaccination for refractory multiple myeloma using patient-specific tumor idiotype protein or idiotype (VDJ)-derived class I-restricted peptides. Br J Haematol 2007; 139(3): 415-24.

[157]   Bol KF, Figdor CG, Aarntzen EH, Welzen ME. Intranodal vaccination with mRNA-optimized dendritic cells in metastatic melanoma patients. OncoImmunology 2015; 4(8): e1019197.

[158]   Schuler G, Schuler-Thurner B, Steinman RM. The use of dendritic cells in cancer immunotherapy. Curr Opin Immunol 2003; 15: 138-47.

[159]   Kim TW, Hung CF, Ling M, Juang J, He L, Hardwick JM, *et al.* Enhancing DNA vaccine potency by coadministration of DNA encoding antiapoptotic proteins. J Clin Invest 2003; 112: 109-17.

[160] Pajtasz-Piasecka E, Indrová M. Dendritic cell-based vaccines for the therapy of experimental tumors. Immunotherapy 2010; 2: 257-68.

[161] Iwata-Kajihara T, Sumimoto H, Kawamura N, Ueda R, Takahashi T, Mizuguchi H, *et al.* Enhanced cancer immunotherapy using STAT3-depleted dendritic cells with high Th1-inducing ability and resistance to cancer cell derived inhibitory factors. J Immunol 2011; 187: 27-36.

[162] Kaneno R, Shurin GV, Tourkova IL, Shurin MR. Chemomodulation of human dendritic cell function by antineoplastic agents in low noncytotoxic concentrations. J Transl Med 2009; 7: 58.

[163] Montelli Tde C, Peraçoli MT, Rogatto SR, Kaneno R, do Prado CH, Rocha Pde M. Genetic and modifying factors that determine the risk of brain tumors. Cent Nerv Syst Agents Med Chem 2011; 11(1): 8-30.

[164] Shevach EM. Fatal attraction: tumors beckon regulatory T cells. Nat Med 2004; 10: 900-1.

[165] Chaput N, Louafi S, Bardier A, Charlotte F, Vaillant JC, Ménégaux F, *et al.* Identification of CD8+CD25+Foxp3+ suppressive T cells in colorectal cancer tissue. Gut 2009; 58(4): 520-9.

[166] Bonertz A, Weitz J, Pietsch DH, Rahbari NN, Schlude C, Ge Y, *et al.* Antigen-specific Tregs control T cell responses against a limited repertoire of tumor antigens in patients with colorectal carcinoma. J Clin Invest 2009; 119(11): 3311-21.

[167] Brahmer JR, Tykodi SS, Chow LQ, Hwu WJ, Topalian SL, Hwu P, *et al.* Safety and activity of anti-PD-L1 antibody in patients with advanced cancer. N Engl J Med 2012; 66(26): 2455-65.

[168] Foss FM. DAB389 IL-2 (ONTAK): a novel fusion toxin therapy for lymphoma. Clin Lymphoma 2000; 1: 110-6.

[169] Lutsiak ME, Semnani RT, De Pascalis R, Kashmiri SV, Schlom J, Sabzevari H. Inhibition of CD4(+)25+ T regulatory cell function implicated in enhanced immune response by low-dose cyclophosphamide. Blood 2005; 105: 7-2862.

[170] Le DT, Uram JN, Wang H, Bartlett BR, Kemberling H, Eyring AD, *et al.* PD-1 Blockade in Tumors with Mismatch-Repair Deficiency. N Engl J Med 2015; 372(26): 2509-20.

[171] Ji RR, Chasalow SD, Wang L, Hamid O, Schmidt H, Cogswell J, *et al.* An immune-active tumor microenvironment favors clinical response to ipilimumab. Cancer Immunol Immunother 2012; 61(7): 1019-31.

[172] Tumeh PC, Harview CL, Yearley JH, Shintaku IP, Taylor EJ, Robert L, *et al.* PD-1 blockade induces responses by inhibiting adaptive immune resistance. Nature 2014; 515(7528): 568-71.

[173] Le DT, Lutz E, Uram JN, Sugar EA, Onners B, Solt S, *et al.* Evaluation of ipilimumab in combination with allogeneic pancreatic tumor cells transfected with a GM-CSF gene in previously treated pancreatic cancer. J Immunother 2013; 36(7): 382-9.

[174] O'Hara A, Shanahan F. The gut flora as a forgotten organ. EMBO Rep 2006; 7: 688-93.

[175] Sun J, Chang E. Exploring gut microbes in human health and disease: pushing the envelope. Genes Dis 2014; 1: 132-9.

[176] Ivanov II, Honda K. Intestinal commensal microbes as immune modulators. Cell Host Microbe 2012; 12(4): 496-508.

[177] Boleij A, Tjalsma H. Gut bacteria in health and disease: a survey on the interface between intestinal microbiology and colorectal cancer. Biol Rev Camb Philos Soc 2012; 87: 701-30.

[178] Vindigni SM, Zisman TL, Suskind DL, Damman CJ. The intestinal microbiome, barrier function, and immune system in inflammatory bowel disease: a tripartite pathophysiological circuit with implications for new therapeutic directions. Therap Adv Gastroenterol 2016; 9(4): 606-25.

[179] Iida N, Dzutsev A, Stewart CA, Smith L, Bouladoux N, Weingarten RA, *et al.* Commensal bacteria control cancer response to therapy by modulating the tumor microenvironment. Science 2013;

342(6161): 967-70.

[180] Viaud S1. The intestinal microbiota modulates the anticancer immune effects of cyclophosphamide. Science 2013; 342(6161): 971-6.

[181] Sivan A, Corrales L, Hubert N, Williams JB, Aquino-Michaels K, Earley ZM, *et al.* Commensal Bifidobacterium promotes antitumor immunity and facilitates anti-PD-L1 efficacy. Science 2015; 350(6264): 1084-9.

[182] Vétizou M, Pitt JM, Daillère R, Lepage P, Waldschmitt N, Flament C, *et al.* Anticancer immunotherapy by CTLA-4 blockade relies on the gut microbiota. Science 2015; 350(6264): 1079-84.

CHAPTER 2

Adjudin - A Male Contraceptive with Anti-Cancer, Anti-Neuroinflammation and Anti-Ototoxicity Activities

Yan-ho Cheng[1,2]**, Weiliang Xia**[3]**, Xiang Xiao**[1,4]**, Elizabeth Tang**[1]**, Haiqi Chen**[1]**, Qing Wen**[1]**, Ying Gao**[1]**, Dolores Mruk**[1]**, Bruno Silvestrini**[5] **and C. Yan Cheng**[1,*]

[1] *The Mary M. Wohlford Laboratory for Male Contraceptive Research, Center for Biomedical Research, Population Council, 1230 York Ave, New York, New York 10065, USA*

[2] *Oncology and Hematology Program, Department of Medicine, Westchester Medical Center, Valhalla, New York 10595, USA*

[3] *State Key Laboratory of Oncogenes and Related Genes, Renji-Med X Stem Cell Research Center, Ren Ji Hospital; School of Biomedical Engineering, Shanghai Jiao Tong University, Shanghai, China*

[4] *Department of Reproductive Physiology, Zhejiang Academy of Medical Sciences, Hangzhou 310013, China*

[5] *S.B.M. Srl Pharmaceuticals, Rome, Italy*

Abstract: Adjudin, 1-(2,4-dichlorobenzyl)-*1H*-indazole-3-carbohydrazide, is an indazole-based compound and a testis-specific adherens junction disruption inducer. Adjudin is also an analog of the anticancer drug lonidamine. Studies have shown that adjudin is an effective male contraceptive in rats, rabbits, and beagle dogs. Adjudin is known to exert its effects primarily at the testis-specific actin-rich adherens junction known as ectoplasmic specialization (ES), most notably in the adluminal compartment called apical ES at the Sertoli-spermatid (step 8-19) interface in adult rat testes. Similar ultrastructures of apical ES are also found in the mouse, dog and human testes.

Specifically, adjudin has been shown to perturb the organization of actin microfilament bundles at the ES, which in turn, perturbs adhesion protein complexes that utilize F-actin for attachment.

The net result thus perturbs spermatid adhesion to the Sertoli cell in the testis, leading to massive exfoliation of elongated/elongating spermatids, to be followed by round spermatids, spermatocytes and differentiated spermatogonia, but not undifferentiated spermatogonia. This thus induces reversible infertility in rats, rabbits and beagle dogs due to the loss of germ cells in the seminiferous epithelium; and undifferentiated

---

[*] **Corresponding author C. Yan Cheng:** The Mary M. Wohlford Laboratory for Male Contraceptive Research, Center for Biomedical Research, Population Council, 1230 York Ave, New York, 10065, USA; Tel: 212 237 8738; Fax: 212 327 8733; E-mail: Y-Cheng@popcbr.rockefeller.edu, ccheng@rockefeller.edu

Atta-ur-Rahman & M. Iqbal Choudhary (Eds.)

spermatogonia gradually replace all classes of germ cells *via* spermatogenesis, making the adjudin treated animals fertile again. Recent studies, however, have shown that adjudin also possesses biological activities to disrupt cancer growth and tumorigenesis. It also interferes with neuroinflammation by reducing ischemia-induced microglial activation in mice. Furthermore, adjudin protects rodent cochlear hair cells against gentamicin-induced ototoxicity *via* the SIRT3-ROS (SIRT3 also known as Sirtuin 3, silent mating type information regulation 3 homolog (a mitochondria NAD-dependent protein deacetylase)-reactive oxygen species) pathway. In this review, we summarize some of the recent findings, in particular the likely mechanism(s) of action, regarding the multiple biological activities of adjudin, illustrating this potential male contraceptive has other added health benefits, such as preventing cancer growth and development. Furthermore, its use as novel anti-cancer drug is an area of research that can be further explored. Using a multidrug nanocarrier to deliver adjudin, in combination with other anti-cancer drug(s) (*e.g.* doxorubicin), this approach has been used successfully to eradicate drug resistant cancer cells.

Keywords: Adjudin, Anti-cancer drug, Anti-inflammatory drug, Anti-ototoxicity drug, Male contraceptive, Spermatogenesis, Testis.

INTRODUCTION

Design of optimal chemotherapy to treat different human cancers is a rapidly changing field [1 - 3]. Interestingly, the use of "old" drugs, either alone or in combination with other drug(s), intended for treating other illnesses has shown to be promising for cancer therapy. Also, this approach saves time by reducing hurdles for clinical trials. For instance, the use of metformin (an anti-diabetic drug) or insulin in cancer therapy [4, 5], chloroquine (an anti-malarial and anti-rheumatoid drug) in treating glioma [6, 7], and silibinin (a liver detoxifying drug) in cancer therapy [8] have illustrated that the use of some "old" drugs save time, efforts and resources for development. This is because their safety has already been proven in earlier clinical trials for intended applications. Adjudin, a second generation indazole-based compound, closely related to the anti-cancer drug lonidamine, has been investigated as a potential male contraceptive [9 - 11]. Studies in the 1970s and 1980s have shown that indazole-based compounds also possess potent anti-spermatogenic activities by targeting mitochondria found in germ cells [12 - 14], perturbing germ cell energy metabolism [15, 16]. Subsequent studies have shown that lonidamine also possesses potent activity to perturb cancer cell metabolism by acting as a mitochondrial hexokinase inhibitor [15, 17, 18]. In fact, lonidamine by itself is a new class of anti-cancer drug by blocking tumor cell energy metabolism instead of an anti-mitotic drug [19, 20]. Earlier studies have shown that adjudin, 1-(2,4-dichlorobenzyl)-1H-indazole-3-carbo-hydrazide, formerly called AF-2364, is less toxic based on both acute toxicity and subchronic toxicity tests [9] when compared to lonidamine. This thus raises the expectation that adjudin may have similar anti-cancer activity as of lonidamine, but considerably reduced cytotoxicity. Indeed, adjudin is known to possess anti-proliferation activity on cancer cells *in vitro*, and also on lung and prostate tumors inoculated in athymic nude mice in *in vivo* by shrinking the solid tumors considerably [21]. A recent report has also demonstrated the use of a multi-drug nanocarrier approach using adjudin and doxorubicin to treat drug-resistant cancer cells [22], illustrating the potential of using adjudin as an anti-cancer drug. In this Chapter, we review data regarding the mechanism of action of adjudin in perturbing spermatogenesis in the testis. We also briefly summarize findings that investigate its mechanism of action in cancer cells. Furthermore, adjudin is known to possess anti-inflammatory and anti-ototoxicity activities. Collectively, this information will provide a solid basis to better understand the different mechanisms of action of adjudin in mammalian cells and tissues (Fig. **1**). This information should appeal to cancer biologists, and investigators interested in illnesses in the brain such as Alzheimer's disease, as well as reproductive biologists.

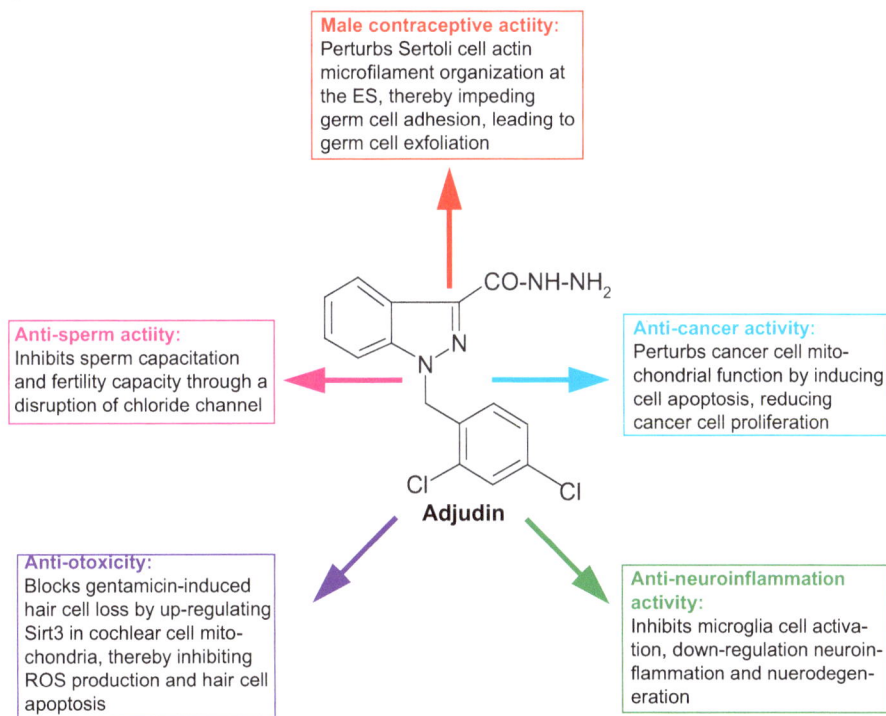

Fig. (1). Adjudin and its various activities in rodents based on studies *in vitro* and/or *in vivo*. Structural formula of adjudin, 1-(2,4-dichlorobenzyl)-*1H*-indazole-3-carbohydrazide, illustrating adjudin, similar to lonidamine, is an indazole-based drug but without the toxicity of lonidamine. Based on recent studies using various *in vitro* and *in vivo* models as discussed in text, adjudin is now known to be a reversible male contraceptive in rats and rabbits. Interestingly, adjudin also possesses anti-cancer, anti-neuroinflammation/anti-neurodegeneration, and anti-hearing loss activity. These other potential health benefits provide additional incentives to explore this drug as a male contraceptive in humans.

INDAZOLE-RING CONTAINING ANTI-CANCER DRUGS

Lonidamine

Lonidamine, 1-(2,4-dichlorobenzyl)-1H-indazole carboxylic acid, is one of the lead indazole-based compounds synthesized in the 1970s of a new class of anti-cancer drugs without the usual anti-mitotic activity of most anti-cancer drugs [20]. Instead, lonidamine is a mitochondria-targeting drug by acting as a potent inhibitor of mitochondria-bound hexokinase by depriving energy supply to cancer cells, causing apoptosis of tumor cells [23, 24]. Lonidamine is also effective in blocking tumor growth by impeding mitochondria function by blocking electron transports, such as hydrogen ions, across the inner membrane of mitochondria, thereby blocking oxidative phosphorylation and reducing mitochondrial membrane potential and energy metabolism, leading to apoptosis even in doxorubicin-resistant cancer cells [15, 25 - 27]. The clinical value of lonidamine was shown in both phase II and phase III trials against a variety of solid tumors [28]. Interestingly, lonidamine was found to have poor clinical efficacy when used alone, yet it was highly effective when used in combination with other anticancer drugs, such as diazepam and paclitaxel when explored for its use for late-stage cancer patients [29 - 31]. Lonidamine was also found to possess anti-spermatogenetic activity by causing exfoliation of germ cells following treatment of rodents at ~100 mg/kg b.w. by oral gavage [12, 32] in initial animal studies. This effect was mediated by lonidamine-induced Sertoli cell injury wherein extensive vacuolization was detected in lonidamine treated rats, as well as reducing Sertoli cell aromatase activity, impeding the production of estradiol-17β in the testis [33]. Studies have shown that testis function is regulated, at least in part, under the influence of an optimal balance of testosterone and estradiol-17β, with aromatase that converts testosterone or estradiol-17AY, acts as a crucial modulator [34, 35]. Earlier reports using an ERα (estrogen receptor α) knockout (KO) mouse model has shown that estradiol-17β is important to regulate luminal fluid resorption of efferent ductules *via* its effect on the ion transporters and aquaporin water channels in efferent ductules [36 - 38]. These ERKO mice had severe luminal fluid backed up in the rete testis and seminiferous tubules, leading to eventual degeneration of seminiferous epithelium in tubules, to be followed by testis atrophy and infertility [34, 39, 40]. Recent studies have also shown that estradiol-17β is necessary for the maintenance of spermatogenesis in particular the development and final maturation of spermatozoa and transcriptional regulation [34, 41, 42]. However, it remains to be determine if adjudin, an analog of lonidamine, has any disruptive effects on the aromatase activity of Sertoli cells or germ cells since germ cells are known to express relatively high level of aromatase in the testis [43]. Interestingly, lonidamine has no apparent disruptive effects on Sertoli cell aerobic glycolysis and energy metabolism [44], but it is capable of disrupting mitochondrial membrane potential of germ cells, leading to mitochondrial degeneration, causing maturation arrest of spermatids during spermiogenesis in the rat testis [16]. Thus, lonidamine and its related indazole compounds, such as tolnidamine and adjudin, have become a new class of anti-spermatogenetic drugs. For instance, these drugs exert their effects not on germ cells but to induce reversible Sertoli cell injury, causing reversible infertility in male rodents and rabbits [10 - 12, 45].

Adjudin

Male Contraceptive Activity

Studies in the last two decades have demonstrated the anti-spermatogenetic effect of adjudin in which it induces germ cell exfoliation from the testis efficiently [10, 11, 46]. The initial study has shown that adjudin (formerly called AF-2364) induces the expression of an apical ES-based signaling protein known as testin [47, 48] by several orders of magnitude, as much as 50-fold, when assessed by gene profiling approach [49] besides PCR and immunoblotting [48, 50], analogous to another adjudin analog called gamendazole and H2-gamendazole [51, 52]. These initial findings thus suggest that adjudin exerts its effects primarily or initially at the apical ES which is the only anchoring device between elongating/elongated spermatids (step 8-19) and the Sertoli cell in the seminiferous epithelium [50, 53]. Subsequent studies have shown that adjudin rapidly induces disruption of the apical ES, as short as ~6 hr when elongating/elongated spermatids begin to detach from the epithelium in 50% of the seminiferous tubules examined, to be followed by round spermatids and spermatocytes which takes as much 3- and 6.5-day, respectively, for 50% of tubules display signs of their exfoliation [54, 55]. These findings thus prompted us to perform a two decades long study to better understand the biology of spermatid adhesion in the testis, focusing on the structural and functional aspect of ES in the testis [56 - 59]. These findings also formed the basis for us to identify the molecular target of adjudin in the testis, illustrating adjudin specifically binds to testin and actin microfilaments at the ES [60]. Interestingly, while the apical and basal ES (note: basal ES is at the Sertoli cell-cell interface near the basement membrane in the epithelium, which together with the tight junction (TJ) create the blood-testis barrier (BTB)) share almost identical ultrastructural features in the testis wherein bundles of actin microfilaments are sandwiched in-between the apposing Sertoli-spermatid and Sertoli-Sertoli cell plasma membranes, respectively, and cisternae of endoplasmic specialization [61 - 64]. The apical ES at the spermatid-Sertoli cell interface is more sensitive to adjudin treatment [55]. For instance, following a single dose of adjudin (50 mg/kg b.w., by oral gavage), it takes just ~6 hr for adjudin to induce degeneration of apical ES to elicit spermatid loss from the seminiferous epithelium [54, 65]. A study by electron microscopy has shown that adjudin effectively induces defragmentation of actin microfilament bundles at the apical ES [66]. Truncation of actin microfilaments thus perturbs spermatid polarity in which the heads of developing spermatids no longer strictly point toward the basement membrane and are arranged randomly across the seminiferous epithelium [66]. Interestingly, it takes at least two weeks before basal ES/BTB is disrupted, making the barrier "leaky" [57, 65]. The delayed response of the basal ES compared to apical ES following a single oral dose of adjudin at 50 mg/kg b.w. is likely due to the presence of two arrays of actin filament bundles at the basal ES, found on both sides of the adjacent Sertoli cells that reinforce the barrier function at the BTB *vs.* a single array of actin filament bundles at the apical ES to confer spermatid adhesion. As it is logical to conceive that it takes longer for adjudin to disrupt two arrays of actin filament bundles at the basal ES compared to just a single array of actin filament bundles at the apical ES. In this context, it is of interest to note that it remains to be determined if adjudin would have any effects on Sertoli cell aerobic glycolysis and energy metabolism, and if, like lonidamine, it would perturb germ cell mitochondrial function.

Anti-cancer Activity

Similar to lonidamine, adjudin is a drug recently shown to display anti-cancer activity against a number of cancer cell lines with potency better than lonidamine, usually by ~3-4 fold, based on its IC_{50} by blocking cell proliferation in adenocarcinoma cells of human lung, stomach, pancreas, breast, and ovary, as well as human glioma cells and prostate cancer cells [21]. This anti-proliferation activity is dose-dependent. Adjudin also exerts its effects by inducing cancer cell apoptosis *via* the caspase-3-dependent pathway, and perturbing mitochondrial function by down-regulating mitochondrial membrane potential and disrupting electron transport [21]. This, in turn, reduces intracellular ATP level considerably [21]. These findings are also consistent with an earlier report that adjudin induces a considerable loss of sperm mitochondrial membrane potential, and interferes with energy production in germ cells [67], similar to the disruptive effects of lonidamine on mitochondrial function [25 - 27]. These findings thus support the notion that determined if adjudin is a mitochondria hexokinase inhibitor like lonidamine. Based on the anti-cancer activity shown in standard assays *in vitro*, adjudin is also shown to reduce lung and prostate carcinoma cell growth *in vivo* considerably using lung and prostate tumor models on athymic nude mice [21]. An interesting observation is that adjudin is effective to inhibit proliferation of A549 (human lung adenocarcinoma cells) cells by causing these cells to undergo apoptosis with an IC_{50} at 63 AμM, (*vs.* lonidamine at 205 AμM). But when adjudin is used in combination with cisplatin, this multi-drug approach can reduce the effective dose of IC_{50} to 15 AμM for adjudin (with cisplatin at 25 AμM), rendering adjudin to become a more effective anti-cancer drug [21]. These findings thus illustrate the synergistic effects of adjudin in chemotherapy in which adjudin is an excellent adjuvant for combination cancer therapy. Indeed, a recent report using a drug conjugation and nanocarrier approach by combination delivery of adjudin and doxorubicin (also known as Adriamycin or Rubex, a common chemotherapeutic drug that exerts its effects by intercalating DNA, with a serious side effect of causing heart damage) is highly effective for the treatment of drug-resistant cancer cells (*e.g.*, MCF-7/ADR cells) when doxorubicin alone was not effective [22]. In brief, doxorubicin is conjugated to adjudin *via* an acid-sensitive covalent hydrazone bond, to be followed by encapsulation of adjudin-doxorubicin conjugates by $DSPE-PEG_{2000}$ (1,2-distearoyl-sn-glycero-3-phosphoethanol-mine-N-(amino(polyethylene glycol)-2000) micelles [22]. These adjudin-doxorubicin conjugated/encapsulated micelles are stable under physiological conditions and rapidly uptake and engulfed by mammalian cells *via* the endocytic pathway, being placed inside the endolysosomes with a moderate acidic environment, escaping the detection of these drugs by the drug transporters (*e.g.*, P-glycoprotein, breast cancer resistant protein (BCRP)) [68]. This thus accelerates hydrolysis of the hydrazone bond, releasing adjudin and doxorubicin as two effective drug entities to exert their effects to cause apoptosis of drug-resistant cancer cells [22]. Additionally, the use of this nanocarrier multi-drug approach is more effective to induce apoptosis of MCF-7/ADR cells by reducing cell viability using adjudin-doxorubicin/DSPE-PEG2000 *vs.* adjudin or doxorubicin alone [22].

Anti-inflammatory/Anti-neurodegeneration Activities

In the brain, microglia are the resident macrophages that are involved in brain development, repair, inflammation and multiple brain disorders [69 - 72]. Studies have shown that microglial activation causes inflammation in the CNS (central nervous system), and chronic inflammation is one of the major contributing factors to the onset and pathogenesis of brain disorders including Alzheimer's disease, Parkinson disease, depression, schizophrenia and multiple sclerosis [73 - 77]. When microglia are activated, they produce several proinflammatory mediators, which include cytokines (*e.g.*, TNFα, IL-1β), chemokines, Toll-like receptors (*e.g.*, TLR-2, TLR-4), reactive oxygen species (ROS), nitric oxide (NO) and prostaglandin E2 (PGE2), which are neurotoxic when neurons in the brain are exposed chronically, leading to different diseases of the brain as noted above [72, 78]. In this context, it is of interest to note that many indazole-based compounds, most notably bindarit and benzydamine are also non-steroidal anti-inflammatory drugs (NSAID) by inhibiting the production of PGE2, NO, cytokines and/or chemokines in mammalian cells [79 - 83]. In fact, indazole derivatives (*e.g.*, bindarit) have been explored as anti-inflammatory drugs for studies both *in vitro* and *in vivo*, such as by inhibiting NF-κB activation [82, 84 - 86]. A recent study has shown that adjudin inhibited LPS (lipopolysaccharide)-induced release of IL-6, and also down-regulated the expression of IL-6, IL-1β, and TNF-α in BV2 microglia cells *in vitro* [87]. Adjudin also inhibited NI-κB p65 nuclear translocation and DNA binding activity and ERK phosphorylation in BV2 microglia cells *in vitro* [87]. A permanent middle cerebral artery occlusion (pMCAO) mouse model that mimics ischemia-induced chronic brain inflammation with microglial activation as manifested by a surge in CD11b expression [87], which is a known marker of microglial activation in CNS diseases [88], has also been used to examine the role of adjudin *in vivo*. Treatment of pMCAO mice with adjudin was found to reduce brain edema, associated with attenuated neurological defects following ischemia [87]. There is evidence suggesting that activated microglia secrete considerably more metalloproteinases (MMPs) in the brain following stroke [89], thereby causing extensive tissue damage. It is likely that adjudin blocks brain-edema by inhibiting microglia-induced brain damage through a reduced production of MMPs. This possibility which should be carefully evaluated in future studies. Nonetheless, these observations support the notion that adjudin attenuates neuroinflammation, illustrating its likely protective role in interfering neurodegeneration caused by chronic inflammation mediated by microglial activation.

Anti-ototoxicity Activity

Aging is associated with degeneration of hair cells in the cochlea, leading to irreversible hearing loss [90, 91]. As such, it is important to identify drugs and/or approaches to halt or reduce the pace of hair cell loss during aging or other pathological conditions. Using an established gentamicin-induced hair cell loss model *in vitro*, adjudin was found to block gentamicin-mediated cochlear hair cell damage by up-regulating Sirt3 (silent information regulator 3) in mitochondria of cochlear cells, which in turn inhibited ROS production, attenuating hair cell apoptosis [92]. In this context, it is of interest to note that Sirt3 is a member of the growing family of Sirts (silent information regulators also known as sirtuins which are NAD(+)-dependent protein deacetylases, comprising of Sirt 1 to Sirt7 in which Sirt3, Sirt4 and Sirt5 are restrictively expressed in the mitochondria) proteins whose most notable function is to deacetylate a number of metabolic enzymes in particular glycolysis and the Krebs cycle by altering their activity by mediating responses to stresses in particular calorie restriction and metabolic stress [93] (for reviews, see [94, 95]). This observation was further confirmed by overexpressing Sirt3 in cochlear explants by transfecting lentivirus containing the Sirt3 full-length cDNA. Hair cells overexpressing Sirt3 were found to attenuate gentamicin-induced hair cell loss [92], illustrating the otoprotective effects of adjudin in gentamicin-induced hair cell apoptosis. Hair cells transfected with lentivirus containing Sirt3-specific short hairpin RNA (sh-Sirt3) to knockdown Sirt3 in cochlear explants, treatment of explants with adjudin no longer capable of rescuing gentamicin-induced hair cell damage effectively [92], illustrating adjudin mediated its oto-protective effects through Sirt3. These findings were also confirmed using an *in vivo* animal model using gentamicin to induce hearing loss in mice. Administration of adjudin was found to effectively prevent gentamicin-induced hearing loss in mice based on histological analysis but also electrophysiological analysis such as by quantifying auditory brainstem response (ABR) and compound action potential (CAP) in mice [92]. In short, adjudin offers its ototoxicity protective effects by up-regulating Sirt3 expression and inhibiting ROS production in mitochondria, thereby interfering gentamicin-induced hair cell apoptosis. These findings also illustrate the anti-otoxocity effects of adjudin is mediated through its effects on the mitochondrial Sirt3. It has been reported that Sirt3 stimulates isocitrate dehydrogenase 2, an enzyme that converts $NADP^+$ to NADPH in mitochondria, thereby increasing the ratio of reduced glutathione: oxidizied glutathione and decreasing ROS production [96], which is found to prevent age-related hearing loss under caloric restriction [96]. Subsequent study has shown that Sirt3 exerts its hearing loss protective effects by promoting urea cycle and fatty acid oxidation during dietary restriction [97]. While much work is needed to better define the otoprotective effects of adjudin in gentamicin-induced hearing loss by mediating a surge in Sirt3 expression in hair cells of cochlea. These findings, however, are consistent with other studies in which adjudin exerts one of its effects in the mitochondria by inducing cancer cell apoptosis by altering the metabolic homeostasis of tumor cells [21].

CONCLUDING REMARKS AND FUTURE PERSPECTIVES

In this Chapter, we have highlighted some of the latest findings regarding the mechanism of action of adjudin as a potential anti-cancer drug by inducing cancer cell apoptosis *via* its effects on mitochondrial energy metabolism in cancer cells. It also exerts its effects to block microglia cell activation, the hallmark response of chronic neuroinflammation (and neurodegeneration) that marks the onset of many neurological disorders including Alzheimer's disease and dementia. More important, adjudin also up-regulates Sirt3 in mitochondria of hair cells in cochlea to protect hair cell degeneration using a gentamicin-induced ototoxicity in studies *in vitro* and *in vivo*. Besides its anti-spermatogenic effects in the testis by perturbing the actin microfilament organization in Sertoli cells, thereby perturbing germ cell adhesion most notably elongated/elongating spermatids, causing germ cell exfoliation in adult testes of rats and rabbits. These findings have unequivocally demonstrated the diverse cellular effects of adjudin. Nonetheless, much work is needed to identify if these diverse cellular effects of adjudin are mediated through a common downstream signaling protein (or signaling pathway) or a few inter-related signaling proteins. For instance, studies have shown that Sirt3 blocks ROS-mediated hyperactivation of Akt signaling (for a review, see [94]). Sirt1-mediated deacetylation also regulates Akt binding onto PIP3 (phosphatidylinositol (3,4,5)-triphosphate) - the hallmark of Akt activation through its binding to PIP3 (for reviews, see [94, 98]). Recent studies have shown that Akt1/2 signaling is involved in the mTORC1-mediated effects on actin microfilament organization and the activation of MMP-9 (matrix metalloprotease 9) at the Sertoli cell blood-testis barrier (BTB), making the barrier leaky, which is necessary to promote the transport of preleptotene spermatocytes across the barrier at stage VIII of the epithelial cycle to support spermatogenesis [99 - 101]. In short, it remains to be determined if Akt1/2 and/or MMP-9 activation is also utilized during adjudin-mediated microglia cell activation, cancer cell apoptosis, or hair cell Sirt3 up-regulation in cochlea. Furthermore, deployment of adjudin in combination with other drugs using nanotechnology as an alternative delivery approach should be vigorously investigated. The answer to some of these questions and the expanded studies of nanocarrier approach should be helpful in future studies to unfold the mechanism of action of adjudin *vs.* its health benefits in humans.

CONFLICT OF INTEREST

The authors declares no conflict of interest, financial or otherwise.

ACKNOWLEDGEMENTS

Studies performed in our laboratories were supported by the National Institutes of Health (NICHD R01 HD056034 to C.Y.C., U54 HD029990 Project 5 to C.Y.C.); Ministry of Science and Technology, China (2013CB945604 to W.X.), National Natural Science Foundation, China (31270032 to W.X., 31371176 to X.X.), Shanghai Jiao Tong University Funding (YG2012ZD05 to W.X.), China Qianjiang Talents Program (QJD1502029 to X.X.), and 2016 Science Technology Department of Zhejiang Province Funding (2016F10010 to X.X.). Y.H.C. was supported by a Clinical Oncology/Hematology Fellowship from New York Medical College (Valhalla, NY); E.T., H.C. and Y.G. were supported by University of Hong Kong (HKU, Hong Kong, China) Research Fellowship Awards. Q.W. was supported by fellowships from HKU, Noopolis Foundation (Rome, Italy), Economic Development Council (New York, NY), and Hong Kong Oriental Logistics Ltd (Hong Kong, China), and Hong Kong Baptist University (Hong Kong, China).

REFERENCES

[1]   Lopez JS, Banerji U. Combine and conquer: challenges for targeted therapy combinations in early phase trials. Nat Rev Clin Oncol 2017; 14(1): 57-66.

[PMID: 27377132]

[2]   Shaked Y. Balancing efficacy of and host immune responses to cancer therapy: the yin and yang effects Nat Rev Clin Oncol 2016; 13(10): 611-26.
[http://dx.doi.org/10.1038/nrclinonc.2016.57]

[3]   Yingchoncharoen P, Kalinowski DS, Richardson DR. Lipid-based drug delivery systems in cancer therapy: What is available and what Is yet to come. Pharmacol Rev 2016; 68(3): 701-87.
[http://dx.doi.org/10.1124/pr.115.012070] [PMID: 27363439]

[4]   Ben Sahra I, Le Marchand-Brustel Y, Tanti JF, Bost F. Metformin in cancer therapy: a new perspective for an old antidiabetic drug? Mol Cancer Ther 2010; 9(5): 1092-9.
[http://dx.doi.org/10.1158/1535-7163.MCT-09-1186] [PMID: 20442309]

[5]   Benni JM, Patil PA. Non-diabetic clinical applications of insulin. J Basic Clin Physiol Pharmacol 2016; 27(5): 445-56.
[http://dx.doi.org/10.1515/jbcpp-2015-0101] [PMID: 27235672]

[6]   Geng Y, Kohli L, Klocke BJ, Roth KA. Chloroquine-induced autophagic vacuole accumulation and cell death in glioma cells is p53 independent. Neuro-oncol 2010; 12(5): 473-81.
[PMID: 20406898]

[7]   Munshi A. Chloroquine in glioblastomanew horizons for an old drug. Cancer 2009; 115(11): 2380-3.
[http://dx.doi.org/10.1002/cncr.24288] [PMID: 19326448]

[8]   Zhu XX, Ding YH, Wu Y, Qian LY, Zou H, He Q. Silibinin: a potential old drug for cancer therapy. Expert Rev Clin Pharmacol 2016; 1-8.
[PMID: 27362364]

[9]   Mruk DD, Wong CH, Silvestrini B, Cheng CY. A male contraceptive targeting germ cell adhesion. Nat Med 2006; 12(11): 1323-8.
[http://dx.doi.org/10.1038/nm1420] [PMID: 17072312]

[10]   Cheng CY, Mruk D, Silvestrini B, *et al.* AF-2364 [1-(2,4-dichlorobenzyl)-*1H*-indazole-3-carbohydrazide] is a potential male contraceptive: a review of recent data. Contraception 2005; 72(4): 251-61.
[http://dx.doi.org/10.1016/j.contraception.2005.03.008] [PMID: 16181968]

[11]   Cheng CY. Toxicants target cell junctions in the testis: Insights from the indazole-carboxylic acid model. Spermatogenesis 2015; 4(2): e981485.
[http://dx.doi.org/10.4161/21565562.2014.981485] [PMID: 26413399]

[12]   Corsi G, Palazzo G, Germani C, Scorza Barcellona P, Silvestrini B. 1-Halobenzyl-1H-indazo-e-3-carboxylic acids. A new class of antispermatogenic agents. J Med Chem 1976; 19(6): 778-83.
[http://dx.doi.org/10.1021/jm00228a008] [PMID: 950645]

[13]   De Martino C, Floridi A, Marcante ML, *et al.* Morphological, histochemical and biochemical studies on germ cell mitochondria of normal rats. Cell Tissue Res 1979; 196(1): 1-22.
[http://dx.doi.org/10.1007/BF00236345] [PMID: 421242]

[14]   de Martino C, Malcorni W, Bellocci M, Floridi A, Marcante M. Effects of AF1312 TS and lonidamine on mammalian testis. A morphological study Chemotherapy 1981; 27: 27-42.

[15]   Floridi A, Bellocci M, Paggi M, Marcante M, De Martino C. Changes in the energy metabolism in the germ cells and Ehrlich ascites tumor cells. Chemotherapy 1981; 27: 50-60.
[http://dx.doi.org/10.1159/000238045]

[16]   Floridi A, DeMartino C, Marcante ML, Apollonj C, Scorza Barcellona P, Silvestrini B. Morphological and biochemical modifications of rat germ cell mitochondria induced by new antispermatogenic compounds: studies *in vivo* and *in vitro*. Exp Mol Pathol 1981; 35(3): 314-31.
[http://dx.doi.org/10.1016/0014-4800(81)90015-0] [PMID: 7308411]

[17]   Floridi A, Lehninger AL. Action of the antitumor and antispermatogenic agent lonidamine on electron

transport in Ehrlich ascites tumor mitochondria. Arch Biochem Biophys 1983; 226(1): 73-83.
[http://dx.doi.org/10.1016/0003-9861(83)90272-2] [PMID: 6227286]

[18]   Floridi A, Paggi MG, Marcante ML, Silvestrini B, Caputo A, De Martino C. Lonidamine, a selective
        inhibitor of aerobic glycolysis of murine tumor cells. J Natl Cancer Inst 1981; 66(3): 497-9.
        [PMID: 6937706]

[19]   Caputo A, Silvestrini B. Lonidamine, a new approach to cancer therapy. Oncology 1984; 41 (Suppl.
        1): 2-6.
        [http://dx.doi.org/10.1159/000225878] [PMID: 6371644]

[20]   Silvestrini B, Palazzo G, De Gregorio M. Lonidamine and related compounds. Prog Med Chem 1984;
        21: 110-35.
        [PMID: 6400133]

[21]   Xie QR, Liu Y, Shao J, *et al.* Male contraceptive Adjudin is a potential anti-cancer drug. Biochem
        Pharmacol 2013; 85(3): 345-55.
        [http://dx.doi.org/10.1016/j.bcp.2012.11.008] [PMID: 23178657]

[22]   Li X, Gao C, Wu Y, Cheng CY, Xia W, Zhang Z. Combination delivery of Adjudin and Doxorubicin
        via integrating drug conjugation and nanocarrier approaches for the treatment of drug-resistant cancer
        cells. J Mater Chem B Mater Biol Med 2015; 3(8): 1556-64.
        [http://dx.doi.org/10.1039/C4TB01764A] [PMID: 27182439]

[23]   Sordet O, RA(c)bA(c) C, Leroy I, *et al.* Mitochondria-targeting drugs arsenic trioxide and lonidamine
        bypass the resistance of TPA-differentiated leukemic cells to apoptosis. Blood 2001; 97(12): 3931-40.
        [http://dx.doi.org/10.1182/blood.V97.12.3931] [PMID: 11389037]

[24]   Ravagnan L, Marzo I, Costantini P, *et al.* Lonidamine triggers apoptosis *via* a direct, Bcl-2-inhibited
        effect on the mitochondrial permeability transition pore. Oncogene 1999; 18(16): 2537-46.
        [http://dx.doi.org/10.1038/sj.onc.1202625] [PMID: 10353597]

[25]   Calvino E, Estañ MC, SimA3n GP, *et al.* Increased apoptotic efficacy of lonidamine plus arsenic
        trioxide combination in human leukemia cells. Reactive oxygen species generation and defensive
        protein kinase (MEK/ERK, Akt/mTOR) modulation. Biochem Pharmacol 2011; 82(11): 1619-29.
        [http://dx.doi.org/10.1016/j.bcp.2011.08.017] [PMID: 21889928]

[26]   Li YC, Fung KP, Kwok TT, Lee CY, Suen YK, Kong SK. Mitochondrial targeting drug lonidamine
        triggered apoptosis in doxorubicin-resistant HepG2 cells. Life Sci 2002; 71(23): 2729-40.
        [http://dx.doi.org/10.1016/S0024-3205(02)02103-3] [PMID: 12383880]

[27]   Belzacq AS, El Hamel C, Vieira HL, *et al.* Adenine nucleotide translocator mediates the mitochondrial
        membrane permeabilization induced by lonidamine, arsenite and CD437. Oncogene 2001; 20(52):
        7579-87.
        [http://dx.doi.org/10.1038/sj.onc.1204953] [PMID: 11753636]

[28]   Di Cosimo S, Ferretti G, Papaldo P, Carlini P, Fabi A, Cognetti F. Lonidamine: efficacy and safety in
        clinical trials for the treatment of solid tumors. Drugs Today (Barc) 2003; 39(3): 157-74.
        [http://dx.doi.org/10.1358/dot.2003.39.3.799451] [PMID: 12730701]

[29]   Oudard S, Carpentier A, Banu E, *et al.* Phase II study of lonidamine and diazepam in the treatment of
        recurrent glioblastoma multiforme. J Neurooncol 2003; 63(1): 81-6.
        [http://dx.doi.org/10.1023/A:1023756707900] [PMID: 12814259]

[30]   Milane L, Duan Z, Amiji M. Therapeutic efficacy and safety of paclitaxel/lonidamine loaded EGFR-
        targeted nanoparticles for the treatment of multi-drug resistant cancer. PLoS One 2011; 6(9): e24075.
        [http://dx.doi.org/10.1371/journal.pone.0024075] [PMID: 21931642]

[31]   Pacilio G, Carteni G, Biglietto M, De Cesare M. Lonidamine alone and in combination with other
        chemotherapeutic agents in the treatment of cancer patients. Oncology 1984; 41 (Suppl. 1): 108-12.
        [http://dx.doi.org/10.1159/000225897] [PMID: 6326014]

[32]   Leone MG, Grippa E, Guidolin D, *et al.* Effects of lonidamine on testicular and epididymal proteins in

the rat. Reprod Toxicol 2000; 14(3): 257-63.
[http://dx.doi.org/10.1016/S0890-6238(00)00076-9] [PMID: 10838127]

[33]   Galdieri M, Monaco L, De Martino C. Morphological and biochemical effects of lonidamine on cultured Sertoli cells. Exp Mol Pathol 1984; 41(2): 202-6.
[http://dx.doi.org/10.1016/0014-4800(84)90036-4] [PMID: 6207044]

[34]   Carreau S, Hess RA. Oestrogens and spermatogenesis. Philos Trans R Soc Lond B Biol Sci 2010; 365(1546): 1517-35.
[http://dx.doi.org/10.1098/rstb.2009.0235] [PMID: 20403867]

[35]   ODonnell L, Robertson KM, Jones ME, Simpson ER. Estrogen and spermatogenesis. Endocr Rev 2001; 22(3): 289-318.
[PMID: 11399746]

[36]   Zhou Q, Clarke L, Nie R, *et al*. Estrogen action and male fertility: roles of the sodium/hydrogen exchanger-3 and fluid reabsorption in reproductive tract function. Proc Natl Acad Sci USA 2001; 98(24): 14132-7.
[http://dx.doi.org/10.1073/pnas.241245898] [PMID: 11698654]

[37]   Ruz R, Gregory M, Smith CE, *et al*. Expression of aquaporins in the efferent ductules, sperm counts, and sperm motility in estrogen receptor-alpha deficient mice fed lab chow *versus* casein. Mol Reprod Dev 2006; 73(2): 226-37.
[http://dx.doi.org/10.1002/mrd.20390] [PMID: 16261609]

[38]   Oliveira CA, Carnes K, Franca LR, Hermo L, Hess RA. Aquaporin-1 and -9 are differentially regulated by oestrogen in the efferent ductule epithelium and initial segment of the epididymis. Biol Cell 2005; 97(6): 385-95.
[http://dx.doi.org/10.1042/BC20040078] [PMID: 15850448]

[39]   Hess RA, Bunick D, Lee KH, *et al*. A role for oestrogens in the male reproductive system. Nature 1997; 390(6659): 509-12.
[http://dx.doi.org/10.1038/37352] [PMID: 9393999]

[40]   Hess RA. Estrogen in the adult male reproductive tract: a review. Reprod Biol Endocrinol 2003; 1(52): 52.
[http://dx.doi.org/10.1186/1477-7827-1-52] [PMID: 12904263]

[41]   Carreau S, Wolczynski S, Galeraud-Denis I. Aromatase, oestrogens and human male reproduction. Philos Trans R Soc Lond B Biol Sci 2010; 365(1546): 1571-9.
[http://dx.doi.org/10.1098/rstb.2009.0113] [PMID: 20403870]

[42]   Sinkevicius KW, Laine M, Lotan TL, Woloszyn K, Richburg JH, Greene GL. Estrogen-dependent and -independent estrogen receptorα signaling separately regulate male fertility. Endocrinology 2009; 150(6): 2898-905.
[http://dx.doi.org/10.1210/en.2008-1016] [PMID: 19264877]

[43]   Carreau S, de Vienne C, Galeraud-Denis I. Aromatase and estrogens in man reproduction: a review and latest advances. Adv Med Sci 2008; 53(2): 139-44.
[http://dx.doi.org/10.2478/v10039-008-0022-z] [PMID: 18614433]

[44]   Floridi A, Marcante ML, DAtri S, *et al*. Energy metabolism of normal and lonidamine-treated Sertoli cells of rats. Exp Mol Pathol 1983; 38(1): 137-47.
[http://dx.doi.org/10.1016/0014-4800(83)90105-3] [PMID: 6832337]

[45]   Hu GX, Hu LF, Yang DZ, *et al*. Adjudin targeting rabbit germ cell adhesion as a male contraceptive: a pharmacokinetics study. J Androl 2009; 30(1): 87-93. [eng.].
[http://dx.doi.org/10.2164/jandrol.108.004994] [PMID: 18802200]

[46]   Mruk DD, Cheng CY. Delivering non-hormonal contraceptives to men: advances and obstacles. Trends Biotechnol 2008; 26(2): 90-9.
[http://dx.doi.org/10.1016/j.tibtech.2007.10.009] [PMID: 18191256]

[47]   Cheng CY, Bardin CW. Identification of two testosterone-responsive testicular proteins in Sertoli cell-enriched culture medium whose secretion is suppressed by cells of the intact seminiferous tubule. J Biol Chem 1987; 262(26): 12768-79.
[PMID: 3624278]

[48]   Cheng CY, Grima J, Stahler MS, Lockshin RA, Bardin CW. Testins are structurally related Sertoli cell proteins whose secretion is tightly coupled to the presence of germ cells. J Biol Chem 1989; 264(35): 21386-93.
[PMID: 2592382]

[49]   Xia W, Mruk DD, Lee WM, Cheng CY. Unraveling the molecular targets pertinent to junction restructuring events during spermatogenesis using the Adjudin-induced germ cell depletion model. J Endocrinol 2007; 192(3): 563-83.
[http://dx.doi.org/10.1677/JOE-06-0158] [PMID: 17332525]

[50]   Cheng CY, Silvestrini B, Grima J, *et al.* Two new male contraceptives exert their effects by depleting germ cells prematurely from the testis. Biol Reprod 2001; 65(2): 449-61.
[http://dx.doi.org/10.1095/biolreprod65.2.449] [PMID: 11466213]

[51]   Tash JS, Chakrasali R, Jakkaraj SR, *et al.* Gamendazole, an orally active indazole carboxylic acid male contraceptive agent, targets HSP90AB1 (HSP90BETA) and EEF1A1 (eEF1A), and stimulates Il1a transcription in rat Sertoli cells. Biol Reprod 2008; 78(6): 1139-52.
[http://dx.doi.org/10.1095/biolreprod.107.062679] [PMID: 18218611]

[52]   Tash JS, Attardi B, Hild SA, Chakrasali R, Jakkaraj SR, Georg GI. A novel potent indazole carboxylic acid derivative blocks spermatogenesis and is contraceptive in rats after a single oral dose. Biol Reprod 2008; 78(6): 1127-38.
[http://dx.doi.org/10.1095/biolreprod.106.057810] [PMID: 18218612]

[53]   Grima J, Silvestrini B, Cheng CY. Reversible inhibition of spermatogenesis in rats using a new male contraceptive, 1-(2,4-dichlorobenzyl)-indazole-3-carbohydrazide. Biol Reprod 2001; 64(5): 1500-8.
[http://dx.doi.org/10.1095/biolreprod64.5.1500] [PMID: 11319158]

[54]   Chen YM, Lee NP, Mruk DD, Lee WM, Cheng CY. Fer kinase/Fer*T* and adherens junction dynamics in the testis: an *in vitro* and *in vivo* study. Biol Reprod 2003; 69(2): 656-72.
[http://dx.doi.org/10.1095/biolreprod.103.016881] [PMID: 12700184]

[55]   Su L, Cheng CY, Mruk DD. Adjudin-mediated Sertoli-germ cell junction disassembly affects Sertoli cell barrier function *in vitro* and *in vivo*. Int J Biochem Cell Biol 2010; 42(11): 1864-75.
[http://dx.doi.org/10.1016/j.biocel.2010.08.004] [PMID: 20713173]

[56]   Cheng CY, Mruk DD. Cell junction dynamics in the testis: Sertoli-germ cell interactions and male contraceptive development. Physiol Rev 2002; 82(4): 825-74.
[http://dx.doi.org/10.1152/physrev.00009.2002] [PMID: 12270945]

[57]   Mruk DD, Cheng CY. Sertoli-Sertoli and Sertoli-germ cell interactions and their significance in germ cell movement in the seminiferous epithelium during spermatogenesis. Endocr Rev 2004; 25(5): 747-806.
[http://dx.doi.org/10.1210/er.2003-0022] [PMID: 15466940]

[58]   Cheng CY, Mruk DD. A local autocrine axis in the testes that regulates spermatogenesis. Nat Rev Endocrinol 2010; 6(7): 380-95.
[http://dx.doi.org/10.1038/nrendo.2010.71] [PMID: 20571538]

[59]   Cheng CY, Mruk DD. An intracellular trafficking pathway in the seminiferous epithelium regulating spermatogenesis: a biochemical and molecular perspective. Crit Rev Biochem Mol Biol 2009; 44(5): 245-63.
[http://dx.doi.org/10.1080/10409230903061207] [PMID: 19622063]

[60]   Mruk DD, Cheng CY. Testin and actin are key molecular targets of adjudin, an anti-spermatogenic agent, in the testis. Spermatogenesis 2011; 1(2): 137-46.

[http://dx.doi.org/10.4161/spmg.1.2.16449] [PMID: 22319662]

[61]   Vogl AW, Vaid KS, Guttman JA. The Sertoli cell cytoskeleton. Adv Exp Med Biol 2008; 636: 186-211.
[http://dx.doi.org/10.1007/978-0-387-09597-4_11] [PMID: 19856169]

[62]   Mruk DD, Cheng CY. Cell-cell interactions at the ectoplasmic specialization in the testis. Trends Endocrinol Metab 2004; 15(9): 439-47.
[http://dx.doi.org/10.1016/S1043-2760(04)00219-X] [PMID: 15519891]

[63]   Wong EWP, Mruk DD, Cheng CY. Biology and regulation of ectoplasmic specialization, an atypical adherens junction type, in the testis. Biochem Biophys Acta 2008; 1778: 692-708.
[http://dx.doi.org/10.1016/j.bbamem.2007.11.006]

[64]   Yan HH, Mruk DD, Lee WM, Cheng CY. Ectoplasmic specialization: a friend or a foe of spermatogenesis? BioEssays 2007; 29(1): 36-48.
[http://dx.doi.org/10.1002/bies.20513] [PMID: 17187371]

[65]   Mok KW, Mruk DD, Lee WM, Cheng CY. Spermatogonial stem cells alone are not sufficient to re-initiate spermatogenesis in the rat testis following adjudin-induced infertility. Int J Androl 2012; 35(1): 86-101.
[http://dx.doi.org/10.1111/j.1365-2605.2011.01183.x] [PMID: 21696392]

[66]   Wong EW, Mruk DD, Lee WM, Cheng CY. Par3/Par6 polarity complex coordinates apical ectoplasmic specialization and blood-testis barrier restructuring during spermatogenesis. Proc Natl Acad Sci USA 2008; 105(28): 9657-62.
[http://dx.doi.org/10.1073/pnas.0801527105] [PMID: 18621709]

[67]   Wang H, Chen XX, Wang LR, Mao YD, Zhou ZM, Sha JH. AF-2364 is a prospective spermicide candidate. Asian J Androl 2010; 12(3): 322-35.
[http://dx.doi.org/10.1038/aja.2010.11] [PMID: 20418891]

[68]   Mruk DD, Su L, Cheng CY. Emerging role for drug transporters at the blood-testis barrier. Trends Pharmacol Sci 2011; 32(2): 99-106.
[http://dx.doi.org/10.1016/j.tips.2010.11.007] [PMID: 21168226]

[69]   Crotti A, Ransohoff RM. Microglial physiology and pathophysiology: Insights from genome-wide transcriptional profiling. Immunity 2016; 44(3): 505-15.
[http://dx.doi.org/10.1016/j.immuni.2016.02.013] [PMID: 26982357]

[70]   Petrelli F, Pucci L, Bezzi P. Astrocyltes and microglia and their potential link with autism spectrum disorders. Front Cell Neurosci 2016; 10(21)

[71]   Wes PD, Sayed FA, Bard F, Gan L. Targeting microglia for the treatment of Alzheimers Disease. Glia 2016; 64(10): 1710-32.
[http://dx.doi.org/10.1002/glia.22988] [PMID: 27100611]

[72]   Hoogland IC, Houbolt C, van Westerloo DJ, van Gool WA, van de Beek D. Systemic inflammation and microglial activation: systematic review of animal experiments. J Neuroinflammation 2015; 12: 114.
[http://dx.doi.org/10.1186/s12974-015-0332-6] [PMID: 26048578]

[73]   Calsolaro V, Edison P. Neuroinflammation in Alzheimers disease: Current evidence and futureA directions. Alzheimers Dement 2016; 12(6): 719-32.
[http://dx.doi.org/10.1016/j.jalz.2016.02.010] [PMID: 27179961]

[74]   Su P, Zhang J, Wang D, *et al.* The role of autophagy in modulation of neuroinflammation in microglia. Neuroscience 2016; 319: 155-67.
[http://dx.doi.org/10.1016/j.neuroscience.2016.01.035] [PMID: 26827945]

[75]   MA1/4ller N, Weidinger E, Leitner B, Schwarz MJ. The role of inflammation in schizophrenia. Front Neurosci 2015; 9: 372.
[http://dx.doi.org/10.3389/fnins.2015.00372] [PMID: 26539073]

[76]   Yirmiya R, Rimmerman N, Reshef R. Depression as a microglial disease. Trends Neurosci 2015; 38(10): 637-58.
[http://dx.doi.org/10.1016/j.tins.2015.08.001] [PMID: 26442697]

[77]   Loane DJ, Kumar A. Microglia in the TBI brain: The good, the bad, and the dysregulated. Exp Neurol 2016; 275(Pt 3): 316-27.
[http://dx.doi.org/10.1016/j.expneurol.2015.08.018] [PMID: 26342753]

[78]   Garden GA, Moller T. Microglia biology in health and disease. J Neuroimmune Pharmacol 2006; 1(2): 127-37.
[http://dx.doi.org/10.1007/s11481-006-9015-5] [PMID: 18040779]

[79]   Foster SJ, Bruneau P, Walker ER, McMillan RM. 2-substituted indazolinones: orally active and selective 5-lipoxygenase inhibitors with anti-inflammatory activity. Br J Pharmacol 1990; 99(1): 113-8.
[http://dx.doi.org/10.1111/j.1476-5381.1990.tb14663.x] [PMID: 2110012]

[80]   Bhatia M, Ramnath RD, Chevali L, Guglielmotti A. Treatment with bindarit, a blocker of MCP-1 synthesis, protects mice against acute pancreatitis. Am J Physiol Gastrointest Liver Physiol 2005; 288(6): G1259-65.
[http://dx.doi.org/10.1152/ajpgi.00435.2004] [PMID: 15691869]

[81]   Zimmerman R, Radhakrishnan J, Valeri A, Appel G. Advances in the treatment of lupus nephritis. Annu Rev Med 2001; 52: 63-78.
[http://dx.doi.org/10.1146/annurev.med.52.1.63] [PMID: 11160768]

[82]   Mora E, Guglielmotti A, Biondi G, Sassone-Corsi P. Bindarit: an anti-inflammatory small molecule that modulates the NFκB pathway. Cell Cycle 2012; 11(1): 159-69.
[http://dx.doi.org/10.4161/cc.11.1.18559] [PMID: 22189654]

[83]   Sironi M, Pozzi P, Polentarutti N, *et al.* Inhibition of inflammatory cytokine production and protection against endotoxin toxicity by benzydamine. Cytokine 1996; 8(9): 710-6.
[http://dx.doi.org/10.1006/cyto.1996.0094] [PMID: 8932982]

[84]   Sommers CD, Thompson JM, Guzova JA, *et al.* Novel tight-binding inhibitory factor-kappaB kinase (IKK-2) inhibitors demonstrate target-specific anti-inflammatory activities in cellular assays and following oral and local delivery in an *in vivo* model of airway inflammation. J Pharmacol Exp Ther 2009; 330(2): 377-88.
[http://dx.doi.org/10.1124/jpet.108.147538] [PMID: 19478133]

[85]   Oh JH, Park EJ, Park JW, Lee J, Lee SH, Kwon TK. A novel cyclin-dependent kinase inhibitor down-regulates tumor necrosis factorα (TNF-α)-induced expression of cell adhesion molecules by inhibition of NF-κB activation in human pulmonary epithelial cells. Int Immunopharmacol 2010; 10(5): 572-9.
[http://dx.doi.org/10.1016/j.intimp.2010.02.004] [PMID: 20156602]

[86]   Guglielmotti A, Aquilini L, DOnofrio E, Rosignoli MT, Milanese C, Pinza M. Bindarit prolongs survival and reduces renal damage in NZB/W lupus mice. Clin Exp Rheumatol 1998; 16(2): 149-54.
[PMID: 9536390]

[87]   Shao J, Liu T, Xie QR, *et al.* Adjudin attenuates lipopolysaccharide (LPS)- and ischemia-induced microglial activation. J Neuroimmunol 2013; 254(1-2): 83-90.
[http://dx.doi.org/10.1016/j.jneuroim.2012.09.012] [PMID: 23084372]

[88]   GonzAlez-Scarano F, Baltuch G. Microglia as mediators of inflammatory and degenerative diseases. Annu Rev Neurosci 1999; 22: 219-40.
[http://dx.doi.org/10.1146/annurev.neuro.22.1.219] [PMID: 10202538]

[89]   del Zoppo GJ, Milner R, Mabuchi T, *et al.* Microglial activation and matrix protease generation during focal cerebral ischemia. Stroke 2007; 38(2) (Suppl.): 646-51.
[http://dx.doi.org/10.1161/01.STR.0000254477.34231.cb] [PMID: 17261708]

[90]   Seymour ML, Pereira FA. Survival of auditory hair cells. Cell Tissue Res 2015; 361(1): 59-63.

[http://dx.doi.org/10.1007/s00441-015-2152-5] [PMID: 25743696]

[91] Brosel S, Laub C, Averdam A, Bender A, Elstner M. Molecular aging of the mammalian vestibular system. Ageing Res Rev 2016; 26: 72-80.
[http://dx.doi.org/10.1016/j.arr.2015.12.007] [PMID: 26739358]

[92] Quan Y, Xia L, Shao J, *et al.* Adjudin protects rodent cochlear hair cells against gentamicin ototoxicity *via* the SIRT3-ROS pathway. Sci Rep 2015; 5: 8181.
[http://dx.doi.org/10.1038/srep08181] [PMID: 25640330]

[93] Hirschey MD, Shimazu T, Goetzman E, *et al.* SIRT3 regulates mitochondrial fatty-acid oxidation by reversible enzyme deacetylation. Nature 2010; 464(7285): 121-5.
[http://dx.doi.org/10.1038/nature08778] [PMID: 20203611]

[94] Pillai VB, Sundaresan NR, Gupta MP. Regulation of Akt signaling by sirtuins: its implication in cardiac hypertrophy and aging. Circ Res 2014; 114(2): 368-78.
[http://dx.doi.org/10.1161/CIRCRESAHA.113.300536] [PMID: 24436432]

[95] Houtkooper RH, Pirinen E, Auwerx J. Sirtuins as regulators of metabolism and healthspan. Nat Rev Mol Cell Biol 2012; 13(4): 225-38.
[PMID: 22395773]

[96] Someya S, Yu W, Hallows WC, *et al.* Sirt3 mediates reduction of oxidative damage and prevention of age-related hearing loss under caloric restriction. Cell 2010; 143(5): 802-12.
[http://dx.doi.org/10.1016/j.cell.2010.10.002] [PMID: 21094524]

[97] Hallows WC, Yu W, Smith BC, *et al.* Sirt3 promotes the urea cycle and fatty acid oxidation during dietary restriction. Mol Cell 2011; 41(2): 139-49.
[http://dx.doi.org/10.1016/j.molcel.2011.01.002] [PMID: 21255725]

[98] Corbi G, Conti V, Russomanno G, *et al.* Adrenergic signaling and oxidative stress: a role for sirtuins? Front Physiol 2013; 4: 324.
[http://dx.doi.org/10.3389/fphys.2013.00324] [PMID: 24265619]

[99] Mok KW, Mruk DD, Silvestrini B, Cheng CY. rpS6 Regulates blood-testis barrier dynamics by affecting F-actin organization and protein recruitment. Endocrinology 2012; 153(10): 5036-48.
[http://dx.doi.org/10.1210/en.2012-1665] [PMID: 22948214]

[100] Mok KW, Chen H, Lee WM, Cheng CY. rpS6 regulates blood-testis barrier dynamics through Arp3-mediated actin microfilament organization in rat sertoli cells. An *in vitro* study. Endocrinology 2015; 156(5): 1900-13.
[http://dx.doi.org/10.1210/en.2014-1791] [PMID: 25714812]

[101] Mok KW, Mruk DD, Cheng CY. rpS6 regulates blood-testis barrier dynamics through Akt-mediated effects on MMP-9. J Cell Sci 2014; 127(Pt 22): 4870-82.
[http://dx.doi.org/10.1242/jcs.152231] [PMID: 25217631]

CHAPTER 3

Manipulating the Tumor Microenvironment: Opportunities for Therapeutic Targeting

Peace Mabeta[1,*] and **Michael S. Pepper**[2]

[1] *Angiogenesis Laboratory, Department of Physiology, Faculty of Health Sciences, University of Pretoria, South Africa*

[2] *Institute for Cellular and Molecular Medicine, Department of Immunology, and SAMRC Extramural Unit for Stem Cell Research and Therapy, Faculty of Health Sciences, University of Pretoria, South Africa*

Abstract: Over the years, there has been a marked change in the modalities of cancer treatment from the use of surgery and radiation therapy as gold standards to the employment of chemotherapy and combination approaches using a variety of modalities. Despite the advances, prognosis generally remains poor due to patients who develop toxicity or become refractory to therapy. The focus of treatment approaches has largely been on eliminating tumor cells. However, recent studies have shown that there is cross talk between tumor cells and their immediate environment, collectively known as the tumor microenvironment (TME).

The TME contributes to certain characteristics of cancer such as hyperproliferation and angiogenesis. As such, the TME has been recognized as an important contributor to cancer progression, cellular invasion and metastatic dissemination. In addition, the TME has been reported to promote adaptive resistance to therapy in a number of cancers.

Herein, we provide a brief overview of the pathophysiology of aspects of the tumor microenvironment. We further review emerging treatment modalities that target this niche and the mechanisms underpinning the efficacy of these therapies.

Keywords: Angiogenesis, Cancer, Chemotherapy, Drug delivery, Endothelial cells, Extracellular matrix, Targeted therapy, Tumor associated fibroblasts, Tumor associated macrophages, Tumor microenvironment.

INTRODUCTION

The key objective of conventional anti-cancer therapies is to eliminate cancer cells [1 - 3]. Despite recent advances in cancer chemotherapy, the efficacy of

* **Corresponding author Peace Mabeta:** Angiogenesis Laboratory, Department of Physiology, Faculty of Health Sciences, University of Pretoria, South Africa; Tel: +27 12 3192339; E-mail: peace.mabeta@up.ac.za

Atta-ur-Rahman & M. Iqbal Choudhary (Eds.)

these treatments has been limited by toxicity and the development of resistance [4, 5].

There is increasing recognition that tumor growth relies on an interplay between tumor cells and their adjacent stroma [6 - 9]. Physiology dictates that the structure and composition of the stroma should support cell function. The stroma also changes dynamically to maintain homeostasis [10]. The tumor stroma has a composition that is different to what would be considered to be physiologically appropriate [11].

The tumor stroma is made up of mesenchymal cells, mainly fibroblasts, immune cells, vascular cells, as well as the extracellular matrix (ECM). Stromal components, together with tumor cells, constitute the tumor microenvironment (TME) [12].

In response to stimulation by various factors including low oxygen levels, tumor cells release molecules which can alter both the structure and the composition of the TME [11, 13]. These changes support tumor perfusion and ultimately enable neoplastic growth and progression; in some instances, they also support metastatic dissemination [13]. The importance of the TME to tumor progression is further reinforced by observations from studies on the influence of the TME on human metastatic cancer cells implanted in different organ environments [14, 15].

These studies have shown that ectopically implanted colon cancer cells do not metastasize, neither regionally nor to distant sites, despite the aggressiveness of the cancer from which the cells were isolated [14]. Yet when the same cells were implanted orthotopically (*i.e.* tumor cells implanted in the tissue of origin), metastatic dissemination occurred. The incidence of metastasis was associated with an increase in the activity of tumor-derived ECM enzymes such as collagenase [14 - 16]. The TME components such as cancer associated fibroblasts (CAF) appear to play a role in ECM remodelling as well as neoplastic expansion [4, 11, 17 - 20].

Cellular components of the TME are influenced by growth factors and enzymes secreted by tumor cells [11]. These cells in turn stimulate angiogenesis and lymphangiogenesis in order to support tumor progression [6, 21]. Also, interaction between various cell populations in the TME have implications for treatment efficacy [22].

THE RATIONALE FOR TARGETING THE TUMOR MICRO-ENVIRONMENT

Conventional chemotherapy remains the mainstay for the treatment of neoplastic disease [1]. This form of therapy has been limited by a number of factors which include poor selectivity and toxicity [13, 23].

Several studies have shown that components of the tumor stroma can interfere with drug extravasation at the tumor site and also promote drug resistance [10, 24]. Therefore, targeted treatment strategies that overcome these barriers within the TME may be of clinical importance.

The objectives of targeted approaches would be i). to realize optimal dosing, ii) to enhance drug accumulation at the tumor site, iii) to reduce non-specific targeting and iv) to reduce adverse effects [20, 25].

MODES OF DRUG TARGETING

Drugs are transported through convection, which is the 'movement of molecules within fluids' as well as through diffusion, which involves the movement of low molecular weight particles along a concentration gradient [26]. Several factors influence the penetration of tumors by drugs [27 - 30]. These factors include hydrostatic pressure, oncotic pressure, electrostatic and concentration gradients between blood vessels and the interstitium, vessel permeability, the surface area over which the exchange will occur and the structure of the ECM [28].

In the context of tumors, due to alterations in both the ECM and the vasculature, drug movement through convection is especially restricted, necessitating the employment of targeted drug delivery approaches. Generally, drug targeting approaches are classified into two categories, passive and active [31].

Passive Targeting

Passive targeting utilizes carriers to achieve drug accumulation at a specific site (Fig. **1**) [31]. This form of targeting seeks to exploit the unique properties of the TME such as the leakiness of the tumor vasculature and dysfunctional fluid drainage due to the abnormal tumor lymphatic vasculature [23, 32].

The carriers commonly used in passive anti-cancer drug targeting include lipid based nanoparticles such as liposomes and micromicelles, polymers and metal (inorganic) carriers such as nanogels and gold nanoparticles respectively [26].

Designed drug carriers with selective extravasation into tumor tissue promote the enhanced permeability and retention (EPR) effect [23]. The selectivity of the carriers for the tumor site relies on the leakiness of the tumor vasculature. Poor lymphatic drainage within the TME further enhances the retention of the therapeutic molecules. For example, nanoparticle-albumin-bound (NAB) technology has been employed as a carrier for taxol in the formulation Abraxane, and was observed to support EPR [33]. The particles are approximately 120 nm in diameter and accumulate in the tumor interstitium [33].

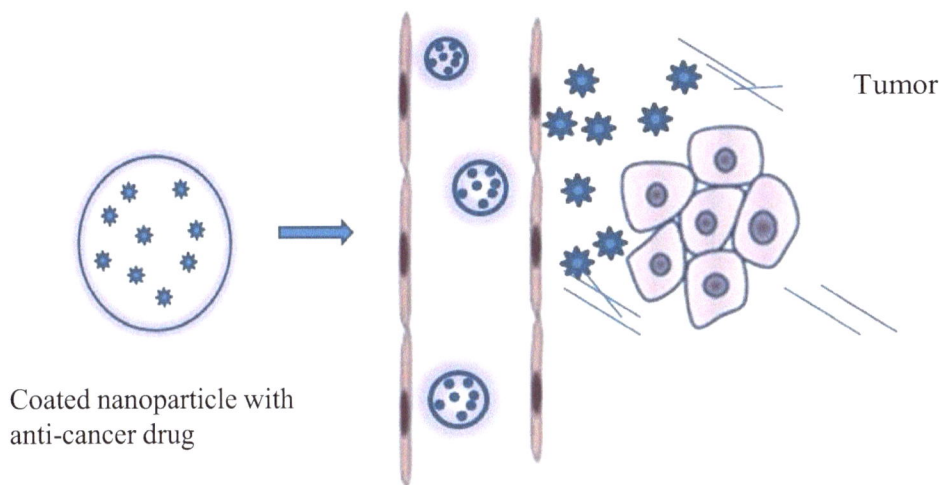

Fig. (1). Passive targeting with a carrier to enhance drug retention at the tumor site. Surface coating is employed to avoid rapid clearance from the blood circulation. Surface coating decreases immunogenicity and reduces uptake by the reticuo-endothelial system.

Abraxane was the first food and drug association (FDA) approved NAB prototype and has been reported to be less toxic than taxol [31, 32]. Another type of carrier, pegylated liposomal nanoparticles was conjugated to docetaxel in the formulation known as Genexol [34]. The formulation has been employed to treat breast, ovarian and lung cancers [31]. The drug conjugate has been shown to be effective as a radiosensitizer in preclinical studies, and is currently undergoing clinical testing [31]. More carriers are being conjugated to standard chemotherapeutics such as doxorubicin and vincristine in order to improve their efficacy (Table **1**).

Table 1. Direct angiogenesis inhibitors employed in passively targeted cancer therapy.

Drug	Indication	Status	Carrier	Reference
Genexol (Taxol)	Lung, breast, pancreatic cancers	Phase II/III	Polymeric micelles	[35, 36]
Abraxane (Taxol)	Metastatic breast cancer	FDA approved	Nanoparticle albumin	[33]
Xyotax (Taxol)	Advanced NSCLC	Phase III	Poly-L-glutamic acid	[31]
Doxil, Myocet (Doxorubicin)	Ovarian, Kaposi sarcoma, metastatic breast cancer	FDA approved	Liposomal nanoparticles	[37, 38]

(Table 1) contd.....

Drug	Indication	Status	Carrier	Reference
Onco-TCS (Vincristine)	Non-Hodgkins, Lymphoma	FDA approved	Liposomal nanoparticles	[39, 39]
DaunoXome (Daunorubicin)	Kaposi sarcoma	FDA approved	Liposomal nanoparticles	[40]

Doxil is an example of liposomal nanoparticles conjugated to doxorubicin [31, 34]. The formulation exploits poor lymphatic drainage in the TME caused by lymph vessel hyperplasia to promote the EPR effect. Doxil has a reduced side-effect profile compared to doxorubicin [31, 34]. It is approved for the treatment of ovarian cancer, Kaposi sarcoma and metastatic breast cancer [34]. The limitation of passive targeting is that not all tumors have the same degree of leakiness that promotes the EPR effect [26].

Active Targeting

Active targeting involves the use of ligand/receptor or stimulus sensitive carriers [23]. The classification of active targeting is further divided into first, second and third order targeting [41]. In first order targeting, there is restricted delivery to a specific tissue site. Second order delivery targets selected cells, while third order targeting entails delivery to intracellular targets [41].

Therapies employed in active targeting of tumor and TME components include monoclonal antibodies and small molecule inhibitors which target cellular communication pathways (Table **2**) [25]. The targeted molecules may be mutated or overexpressed in tumors or in the TME but not in normal tissue [23].

The targeting of vascular endothelial growth factor (VEGF) by bevacizumab is an example of third order active targeting (Fig. **2**). Binding of the targeting mAb to a specific ligand prevents the ligand from binding to its receptor, and in the case of VEGF, prevents the induction of angiogenesis.

Active targeting may employ single molecule therapies (Table **2**) or may be conjugated to combination with antineoplastic drugs [23]. The latter approach has yielded promising results in preclinical studies [42 - 47]. Conjugated cilengitide was shown to be more effective than the unconjugated drug in inhibiting tumor growth in mice [48]. Strategies that combine chemotherapy and AIs have also yielded promising results in clinical studies in patients with glioblastoma [43].

Table 2. Active Targeting antiangiogenic therapies.

Monoclonal Antibodies				
Target	**Drug**	**Status**	**Indications**	**Reference**
EGFR	Cetuximab	FDA approved	Colorectal cancer, head and neck carcinoma	[93]
EGFR	Panitumumab	FDA approved	Colorectal cancer	[93]
VEGF	Bevacizumab	FDA approved	NSCLC, Colorectal cancer	[70, 94]
Her2	Trastuzumab	FDA approved	Her2 positive breast cancer	[44]
Integrin $\alpha v \beta_3$	Vitaxin	Phase II	Metastatic cancers, bone cancer	[42]
Integrin $\alpha v \beta_5$	Celengitide	Phase II	Glioblastoma	[43]
VEGF	Pegatinib	FDA approved	AMD	[72]
Small Molecule Inhibitors				
EGFR	Gefitinib	FDA approved	NSCLC	[45]
EGFR	Erlotinib	FDA approved	NSCLC, pancreatic cancer	[45]
EGFR	Lapatinib	FDA approved	Her2 positive breast cancer	[95]
VEGFR-1,-2,-3, EGFR, PDGFRβ	Sorafenib	FDA approved	Renal cell cancer, hepatocellular carcinoma	[74]
VEGFR-1,-2,-3, PDGFRβ, FLT3, c-KIT	Sunitinib	FDA approved	Renal cell cancer, gastrointestinal stromal tumor	[74]

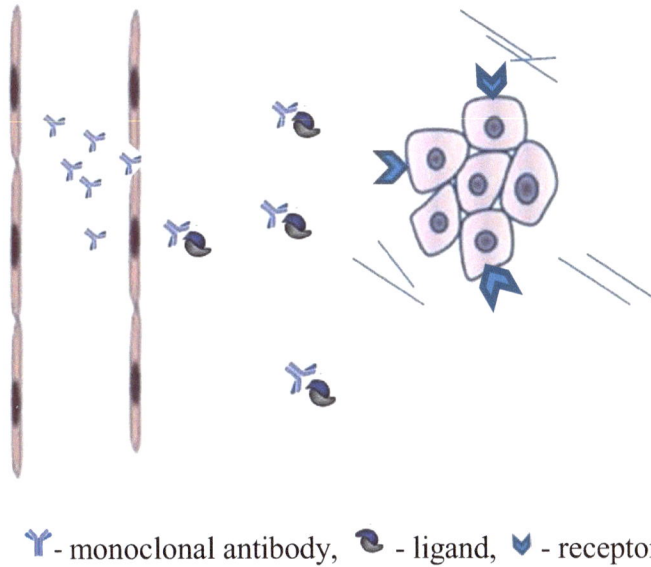

Y- monoclonal antibody, ◔ - ligand, ∨ - receptor

Fig. (2). Active targeting using a neutralizing monoclonal antibody. The monoclonal antibody binds to and sequesters the ligand. This prevents ligand binding to the receptor and ultimately inhibits angiogenesis.

TARGETING COMPONENTS OF THE TME

Different forms of drug targeting have been used to overcome the barriers to anti-cancer treatment that are associated with the multiple components of the TME [7, 9, 48]. These include delivery systems to the ECM, AIs and compounds which target signaling molecules in lymphatic vessels [7].

The Tumor Vasculature

In the adult, the endothelium is relatively quiescent; activation of the vasculature however, occurs during pathological conditions such as cancer [49, 50]. Growing tumors activate an angiogenesis phenotype in response to hypoxia [49]. Angiogenesis is a process of neovessel formation from a pre-existing microvasculature [49, 50].

Several studies have shown that sustained angiogenesis is a hallmark of various malignancies, and that it can be associated with the formation of metastases and a poor prognosis [49, 51, 52]. As such, targeting the tumor vasculature represents an important step in cancer treatment [53].

Recently developed drug delivery systems for the inhibition of angiogenesis exploit the morphological and functional changes associated with the tumor vasculature.

Targeting Morphological Changes to the Tumor Vasculature

The tumor vasculature is characterized by defective architectural organization [49]. Conventional microvascular organization is made up of arterioles, capillaries and venules. The tumor microvasculature does not exhibit a defined vascular hierarchy, but instead the vessels have shared features of different vessel types [4, 54].

The vessels are convoluted, which impairs tumor blood flow and hampers the delivery of anti-cancer drugs [55]. The basal lamina may be absent, and if present, is discontinuous [56, 57]. In addition, support cells, namely, pericytes and smooth muscle cells, are relatively few or absent, thus the vasculature is immature [57, 58]. These attributes make tumor vessels more susceptible to anti-vascular disruption than the more stable and mature 'normal' vasculature.

Tumor blood flow is erratic, and the direction of flow is variable [26]. Also, vessels may be leaky due in part to the presence of fenestrations [59]. Transcapillary filtration is impaired and the net filtration pressure is higher in tumor tissue than in normal tissue, which results in excessive fluid movement into the interstitium [60]. This effect, combined with poor lymphatic drainage, raises the interstitial fluid pressure (IFP) within the tumor stroma. The IFP is high at the center of the tumor and low at the periphery; as a result, effective extravasation of drugs in the central part of the tumor is compromised [61].

Passive targeting employing carriers such as liposomal nanoparticles and gold nanoparticles has exploited this attribute of the tumor vasculature in order to increase the EPR effect.

Some approaches use strategies that lower the tumor IFP. For example AIs that normalize the tumor vasculature have been shown to improve IFP [54, 57, 62, 63]. Lowering the IFP has resulted in improved delivery and efficacy of anti-cancer therapies in pre-clinical tumor models [60].

Another view is that while such approaches enable drug delivery, they limit the extravasation of molecules intended to target the ECM as well as those that work through retention, such as liposomal doxorubicin. This challenge can, however, be overcome by using much smaller carriers, with a diameter of less than 20 nm.

Targeting Functional Changes to the Tumor Vasculature

The functions of the vasculature include transport of nutrients and gases, trans-capillary filtration in various tissues, vascular tone, hemostasis, and hormone trafficking. Endothelial cells provide a non-thrombogenic environment which facilitates the transit of plasma and cellular constituents of blood throughout the vasculature. These functions are affected through growth factors and their receptors, cytokines, and transcription factors such as HIF-1α [49, 64, 65]. These molecules promote vascular tone, prevent thrombosis, and ensure effective transcapillary filtration by playing a role in blood pressure regulation. Furthermore, a balance between pro- and anti-angiogenic factors ensures vascular homeostasis [49, 66].

Some of the molecules that mediate vascular function have been implicated in the pathogenesis of several tumors, and may even be linked to poor prognosis [49, 57, 67]. These molecules include vascular endothelial growth factor (VEGF-A, referred to herein as VEGF) and vascular endothelial growth factor receptors -1 and -2 (VEGFR-1 and VEGFR-2), placental growth factor (PlGF), basic fibroblast growth factor (bFGF), transforming growth factors (TGFs), platelet derived growth factor (PDGF) and its receptor PDGFR, as well as epidermal growth factor (EGF) and its receptor EGFR [49, 57]. An imbalance in factors that promote angiogenesis and those that inhibit it in favor of the former results in the activation of the 'angiogenic switch' that characterizes many cancers [49].

The signaling pathways initiated by these factors and their receptors have been employed in active targeting strategies. Interestingly, these strategies have mainly been focused on AIs rather than vascular disrupting agents (VDA's), perhaps due to the greater success observed thus far in clinical studies with anti-angiogenic strategies.

Angiogenesis Inhibitors

Angiogenesis inhibitors (AIs) are classified as direct or indirect [49]. Direct inhibitors act on vascular endothelial cells and prevent them from proliferating, migrating or invading the ECM. Indirect inhibitors block the expression or effects of proangiogenic factors [49]. Angiogenesis inhibitors and vascular disrupting agents can compromise the delivery of drugs that target tumor cells. As such, normalizing of the tumor vasculature with AIs appears to be a better approach to enhance antineoplasting treatment [62]. Also, monotherapy with AIs such as bevacizumab and sorafenib can lead to disease recurrence.

Bevacizumab was the first AI to receive FDA approval in 2004 [68 - 70]. It is a humanized monoclonal antibody against VEGF and has been employed as single molecule therapy and in combination treatments [68, 70]. However, the use of bevacizumab as monotherapy has been limited by the development of resistance. It is approved for use in combination with other therapies for the treatment of colorectal cancer, metastatic renal cell carcinoma and non-small cell lung carcinoma [71]. Pegaptanib is another mAb which binds VEGF. It is a pegylated aptamer used as an AI in the treatment of age-related macular degeneration (AMD) [72, 73].

Other active targeting antiangiogenic drugs include sorafenib, a multi-kinase inhibitor that targets VEGFR-2, VEGFR-3, platelet derived growth factor receptor (PDGFR) and Raf [74].

Although it has limitations when employed as single agent therapy, sorafenib has been employed in combination with conventional chemotherapy to improve patient outcome [74]. Sunitinib is another multi-kinase inhibitor which targets vascular endothelial growth factor receptor (VEGFR), PDGFR, fms like tyrosine kinase 3 (Flt3), and C-KIT [75, 76]. Other small molecule inhibitors, gefitinib, erlotinib and lapatinib, all target the epidermal growth factor receptor (EGFR) [45, 77].

Approaches aimed at blocking VEGFR-2 have been effective in inhibiting tumor growth in pre-clinical models of cancer, and the blockade of PDGFR signaling improves the efficacy of chemotherapy in mice [54, 78]. In addition, several monoclonal antibodies against receptors such as EGFR and VEGF receptors,-1, -

2, and -3 have been employed successfully in third order active targeting [70, 79].

Active drug delivery systems for inhibiting angiogenesis have also been formulated to target integrins. Integrins are transmembrane protein receptors that mediate cellular attachment to and spreading on the ECM and other cells, and mediate endothelial cell migration during angiogenesis [80]. Integrins can promote resistance to the anti-cancer effects of chemotherapy as well as cancer cell resistance to apoptosis inducers [81, 82].

Studies have showed that the adhesion of cells to fibronectin, a constituent of the ECM, which occurs *via* β1 integrin, contributes to drug resistance [13].

Drug delivery systems that target integrins include celengitide and vitaxin, which target integrins αvβ5 and αvβ3 respectively [42, 43]. Volociximab is another ECM drug delivery system that targets integrins αvβ5 and αvβ3 [83, 84].

Some AIs such as bevacizumab and sorafenib have also been employed in combination strategies with variable results [62, 74, 84, 85]. Three phase III clinical trials testing a combination of the AI, bevacizumab, and chemotherapy in HER2-negative breast cancer showed progression free survival [86, 87]. However, adjuvant treatment with bevacizumab had no effect on overall survival when compared to chemotherapy alone [86 - 88]. Another clinical study demonstrated that adjuvant bevacizumab did not improve disease free survival in triple negative breast cancer [85].

The discontinuation of anti-VEGF treatment has been shown to result in the regrowth of tumor vasculature in both preclinical and clinical studies, and indeed in the clinical setting planned breaks in anti-VEGF therapy have resulted in the re-establishment of the tumor vasculature [75, 89 - 91]. These observations indicate that prolonged and uninterrupted use of this form of targeted therapy may have a better therapeutic effect.

This is further supported by a study showing that prolonged treatment with bevacizumab results in increased overall survival in metastatic colorectal cancer patients [68]. These observations were subsequently validated in a phase III study on metastatic colorectal cancer [71]. On the other hand, treatment breaks and dose reductions may be necessary to limit toxicity, and thus an appropriate balance will need to be established. Perhaps additional targeting beyond VEGF may also yield a better therapeutic outcome.

The fusion protein aflibercept, which binds to and sequesters VEGF and PlGF, when used in combination therapy with fluorouracil, leucovorin and irinotecan (FOLFIRI), improved both progression free survival and overall survival in patients with metastatic colorectal cancer compared to placebo plus FOLFIRI [92].

Targeting the Lymphatic Vasculature

The lymphatic system drains excess fluid from the interstitial space and returns it to the blood circulation. Lymphatic vessels undergo remodeling in cancer [96]. The changes that are associated with the remodeling process include lymphatic hyperplasia, which leads to enlargement of the initial and the collecting lymphatics [21].

In some cancer types, new lymphatic vessels are formed through lymphangiogenesis [21, 96]. These changes enable the metastatic dissemination of tumor cells through the lymphatic system, primarily to lymph nodes.

Lymphatic vessel specific mediators such as VEGF-C and VEGF-D and their receptor (VEGFR-3) modulate the remodeling of tumor lymphatics [96]. Therefore targeting of VEGFC-VEGFR-3 and VEGFD-VEGFR-3 signaling as well as the co-receptor neuropilin 2 may prove effective in restricting lymph node metastasis in preclinical models [96 - 98]. Accordingly, several drugs in various stages of development, including SUYL529 and toloquinol, have been tested against solid tumors in order to restrict lymph-node metastasis [96, 99]. The drugs target different molecules in the VEGFC-VEGFR3 axis as well as VEGFD [99].

VEGFC/D-VEGFR3 signaling involves the activation of CRK I/II, phosphatidylinositol-3 kinase (PI3k) and growth factor receptor binding protein 2 (GRB2), ultimately leading to the activation of C-Jun N-terminal kinase (JNK 1/2), protein kinase B (PKB) and extracellular regulated kinase (ERK 1/2). The activation of these pathways is abrogated by molecules such as YL529 and toloquinol, thus inhibiting lymphangiogenesis [100, 101]. YL529 inhibits VEGFD (Fig. **3**), while toloquinol inhibits VEGFC induced phosphorylation of VEGFR3 [100, 101]. Downstream, the effects of toloquinol are associated with the suppression of ERK 1/2 and PKB [100].

Lymph vessel abnormalities that are characteristic of tumor stroma as well as interstitial fibrosis lead to poor lymphatic drainage which contributes to high interstitial fluid pressure (IFP) in the TME [60]. This ultimately results in restricted extravasation of therapeutic molecules, especially those that are transported by convection [60]. On the other hand, this attribute can be exploited by delivery systems that use diffusion, as the high IFP promotes retention in the tumor interstitium [102].

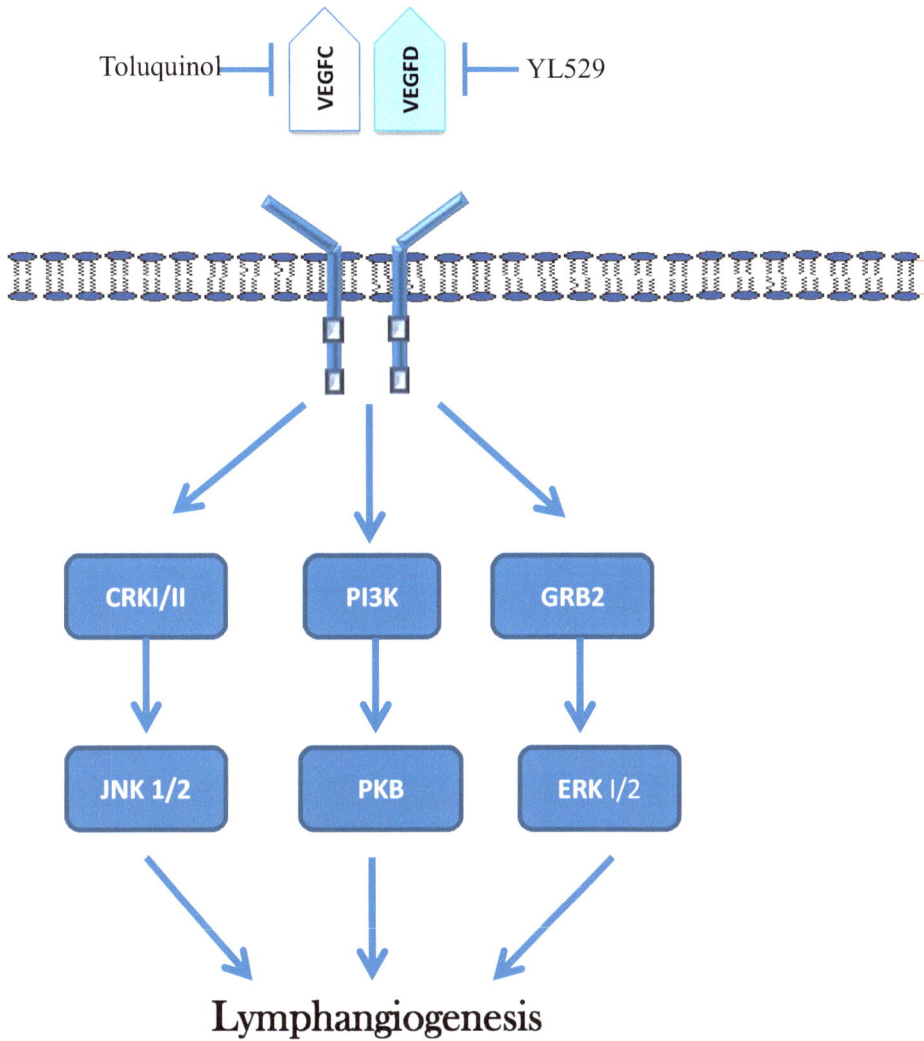

Fig. (3). Schematic representation of the pathways inhibited by therapeutic molecules targeting lymphangiogenic growth factor signaling.

Enhancing Drug Delivery through Targeting of ECM Components

The ECM serves as a scaffold upon and within which cells organize into tissues [103]. It is composed of structural proteins, cell surface receptors and proteases, which all play a role in the mediation of cell-matrix interactions [103]. Such interactions are important for the physiological function of cells as well as for the maintenance of homeostasis. However, during tumorigenesis the protective constraints and homeostatic role of the ECM are overridden by remodeling [7].

The ECM is mainly remodelled in a process involving synthesis and degradation, and the type of ECM formed following remodeling varies in terms of organization and composition in various cancers [4]. The matrix metalloproteinases (MMPs) are a family of zinc dependent endopeptidases which degrade the ECM and thus play an important role in ECM remodeling [26]. In cancer, MMP degradation of the ECM enables EC migration and invasion.

In particular, membrane type 1 MMP (MTI-MMP), which is expressed in EC's associated with the tumor vasculature, contributes to ECM remodeling [26]. Other metalloproteinases associated with the remodeling of the TME include MMP-2 and MMP-9 [80].

The ECM is an important element which determines whether drugs can reach the tumor site [103]. Indeed preclinical data has shown that the abnormal ECM structure in solid tumors provides an obstacle to drug penetration [29]. Inhibitors of MMPs (MMPIs), including membrane-type. 1 matrix metalloproteinase (MT1-MMP), have been tested in various preclinical models for antiangiogenic and antitumor effects [103]. However, clinical trials on MMPIs have largely been unsuccessful [80, 104]. While studies to optimize the targeting of MMPIs have been encouraged, identifying other viable targets in the ECM may have clinical relevance. Another component of the ECM, the matricellular proteins, represents an important role player in the mediation of cell-matrix interactions [105]. The proteins play a functional rather than a structural role in ECM regulation [103, 105]. Matricellular proteins are being explored for therapeutic targeting [106]. Some matrix proteins such as thrombospondin are being assessed for their anticancer properties [107].

Various drug delivery methods have been designed to overcome the challenges presented by the tumor ECM [107, 108]. Thus it was shown that there is a heterogeneous distribution of liposomes in tumor xenografts and that these nanoparticles formed a stagnant perivascular cluster [107]. Other studies have shown that the degradation of ECM components using ECM degrading enzymes such as collagenase improve drug penetration [109, 110]. Also, the hormone relaxin has been used effectively to modify ECM structure [102]. It downregulates the activity of fibroblasts, which are the main source of collagen in the TME, and it also stimulates collagenase activity [108]. While the hormone has enhanced the penetration of doxorubicin into the TME, it was discovered that it also resulted in an increase in the incidence of metastases [108, 111].

Activated CAFs overproduce components of the ECM, including collagen and fibronectin [112]. Activated CAFs also produce factors which stimulate mesenchymal transition during tumorigenesis in which resting fibroblasts are transformed into CAFs [9]. They are the most prominent cells in the tumour stroma in several cancers, especially breast and pancreas [9]. Indeed, increased fibronectin and collagen are synthesized and deposited by activated fibroblasts, and are the major components of the tumor ECM [113].

MESENCHYMAL CELLS AND IMMUNE CELLS

Mesenchymal Cells

Cells of mesenchymal origin have been identified in the TME and have been shown to contribute to be reprogrammed and co-opted into a niche that supports [114]. Mesenchymal stromal/stem cells (MSCs) are recruited by cancer cells from the bone marrow and may also be resident in adipose tissue, such as adipose-derived stem cells (ADSCs) [114].

Excessive adipocity has been associated with an increased risk of cancer development. Adipocyte-derived stem cells, derived from white adipose tissue, can traffic to the tumor tissue [121]. ADSCs produce cytokines and chemokines that further promote tumor progression. The ADSCs also secrete molecules that play an important role in the remodelling of the tumor ECM, such as collagen VI, MMP-2 and MMP-9 [114, 119, 121].

Given their interaction with tumor cells, MSCs have been studied extensively as potential anticancer drug carriers. ADSCs in particular have been tested in clinical trials as stem cell therapy against various conditions including in the suppression of inflammation [115].

In the context of cancer, the targeting of these cells or their use as stem cell therapy has had limited clinical application. Perhaps the success of clinical studies that suppress inflammation might herald promise in the application of ADSCs as rug carriers in cancer treatment.

MSCs engraft into the tumor site and promote tumor growth and progression [117]. The cells also enable tumor cells to evade the immune system [116, 117]. Another cell type that is of mesenchymal origin, fibroblasts, form a significant component of the tumor stroma [118].

Under a physiological setting, fibroblasts promote epithelial quiscence and contribute homeostasis in various organs. *In vitro* in coculture systems, fibrblasts prevent cancer cell growth. However, during tumorigenesis fibroblasts are recruited to the tumor site and they undergo reprogramming to support tumor growth [119]. Fibroblasts recruited to the tumor stroma are known as cancer-associated fibroblasts (CAF) [119]. The fibroblasts are associated with many cancer types such as breast, prostate, pancreatic, lung, gastric, and colorectal. Studies indicate that CAFs contribute to tumor cell proliferation, invasion, and metastasis *via* the secretion of various growth factors, cytokines, chemokines, and ECM degrading proteins [117, 118].

Several CAF-targeted therapies have been tested in pre-clinical models; however, clinical application of these therapies has provided suboptimal results. Immunotherapies that target fibroblast activation protein (FAP), a surface protein overexpressed by CAFs, have been limited by toxicity. Sibrotuzumab, a humanized monoclononal antibody against FAP, failed in phase II clinical trials [119, 120].

Table 3. Drugs targeting immune and mesenchymal cells in cancer treatment.

Drug/Therapy	Target	Cancer Type	Status	Reference
Maraviroc	MSC	Colorectal	Phase 1	[12]
Emactuzumab	TAM	Diffuse type giant tumor	Phase 1	[122]
Nivolumab	CD8+ T cell	Melanoma	Approved	[123]
Ipilimumab	CD8+ T cell	Melanoma	Approved	[124]
Atezolizumab	CD8+ T cell	NSCLC	Phase 2	[12]
IL-1	NK cell	Melanoma, Renal	Phase 1	[12]
Carlumab	MCP-1	Prostate	Phase 2	[125]

Other approaches have been aimed at targeting molecules which activate fibroblasts. The factors that activate fibroblasts include transforming growth factor beta (TGF- β), platelet derived growth factor (PDGF), and basic fibroblast growth factor (bFGF) [7]. Inhibiting these growth factors from activating fibroblasts may block the ECM remodeling that favors tumor growth. In this regard, an anti-TGF-β antibody has been employed successfully to inhibit collagen synthesis in a tumor xenograft [109]. While the targeting of CAFs has presented with challenges, more progress has been observed with therapies that target immune cells (Table **3**).

Immune Cells

Inflammation is a physiological response to tissue damage or infection. It is a beneficial reaction to restore homeostasis and is a self-limiting process [120]. However, when factors that initiate inflammation persist or the mechanisms that resolve inflammation fail, chronic inflammation results, and can lead to cancer [120 - 122]. Also, neoplastic cells produce molecules which attract diverse leukocyte populations that can promote inflammation [121, 122]. These cells include neutrophils, eosinophils, macrophages, mast cells and lymphocytes [120]. These immune cells produce chemicals such as reactive oxygen species (ROS) and cytokines which further promote neoplastic progression [120, 121].

A prominent component of the inflammatory infiltrate is made up of tumor-associated macrophages (TAMs) [121]. Upon recruitment to the tumor site, the macrophages are transformed by factors in the tumor environment to foster tumor progression [8, 121]. TAMs are associated with poor prognosis.

They promote tumor progression by negatively affecting tumor response. Indeed, one of the cytokines produced by TAMs, interleukin 10 (IL-10), blunts the antitumor effects of cytotoxic T-cells [120, 122]. In addition, TAMS produce potent chemoattractants. These chemokines attract myeloid-derived suppressor cells (MDSCs) and dendritic cells (DCs), which further suppress antitumor immunity [122]. Myeloid-derived suppressor cells are also associated with resistance to AI therapy. TAMs produce growth factors such as VEGF, PDGF and FGFs, to promote angiogenesis, and have been implicated in the activation of the 'angiogenic switch' [123]. In addition, TAMs secrete CXCL8, a cytokine which promotes lymphangiogenesis [123]. Given the crucial role these cells play in supporting malignant progression and promoting resistance to anticancer therapy, there has been extensive research into strategies that target the cells.

Some of the modalities in clinical development are listed in Table **3**. Ipilimumab is a monoclonal antibody that targets CD8+ cytotoxic T cells and activates them [124]. Nivolumab CD8+ cytotoxic also activates T cell activation [123]. Another mAb, Carlumab, is in phase II clinical trials. It targets monocyte chemoattractant protein-1 (MCP-1) [125]. MCP-1 is a chemokine that promotes monocyte/ macrophage migration, tumor cell migration and angiogenesis. Thus, neutralizing this chemokine may be of therapeutic benefit.

Developments in Preclinical Strategies

Few of the approaches that target both mesenchymal and immune cells within the TME are in clinical development due in part to challenges of appropriate models to study these cells. PI-3065, which targets T regulatory cells, decreased the growth of tumors in breat and pancreatic cancer mouse models [12].

Another stromal directed therapy targeting mesenchymal cell showing promise in preclinical studies is β-aminopropionitrile (BAPN) [12]. Also, preclinical studies on four murine models of cancer using D-WAT, a peptide which can home to ADSCs, showed that the peptide was able to limit tumor growth [126]. It was also observed in the same study that the presence of an apoptotic domain enhanced the antitumor effect of D-WAT [126]. The findings from these studies also showed unequivocally, that ADSCs promoted tumor growth [126]. Another study has shown a direct relationship between ADSC recruitment to the TME and increased vascularization as well as enhanced tumor progression [127]. Targeting approaches such as with D-WAT may hold promise in anticancer treatment strategies.

CONCLUSION AND FUTURE DIRECTIONS

There is a dynamic bi-directional interaction between tumor cells and the stroma. This was best illustrated in a series of experiments which showed that aggressive tumors transplanted to a non-conducive environment were non-malignant. Mesenchymal, immune and endothelial cells appear to be reprogrammed and co-opted into a niche that supports neoplastic expansion. Of the various components of the TME, extensive research has been undertaken on targeting the tumor vasculature, and several molecules have been tested in clinical trials. The clinical application of modalities that target other stromal components, including immunotherapies, has been limited.

In the context of angiogenesis, VEGF is indispensable for the initiation of the 'angiogenic switch'. However, a diverse array of chemokines, cytokines and growth factors are secreted by tumor cells and they play a crucial role not only in inducing tumor angiogenesis, but also in remodeling the stroma.

Studies further revealed that these factors ultimately promote tumor progression and may also facilitate the emergence of drug resistance. These observations underscore the importance of therapeutic targeting the TME.

It is not surprising that single-molecule therapy with drugs such as Bevacizumab which target VEGF has been associated with the development of resistance, largely due to compensatory mechanisms that develop to overcome the blockade. Modalities that target multiple components of the TME are thus necessary. In addition, advanced drug delivery systems can benefit TME targeting. A mAb against VEGF which was coated to prolong circulation time, Pegaptanib, has been approved for therapeutic anti-angiogenesis in AMD. This may pave the way for the future development of surface coated aptamers for AIs targeting the tumor vasculature.

Prolonged administration of AIs such as Bevacizumab leads to the development of toxicity, while the cessation of treatment is associated with disease recurrence. The development of engineered systems that enable controlled sustained release may be of clinical benefit. Finally, combination approaches that target the TME that are delivered using novel carriers may translate into an improvement in overall patient survival as well as improved quality of life.

CONFLICT OF INTEREST

The authors declares no conflict of interest, financial or otherwise.

ACKNOWLEDGEMENTS

The authors are supported by the National Research Foundation. Work in the lab of MSP is also funded by the South African Medical Research Council (University Flagship and Stem Cell Extramural Unit), and the National Health Laboratory Services Research Trust.

REFERENCES

[1] Blansfield JA, Caragacianu D, Alexander HR III, *et al.* Combining agents that target the tumor microenvironment improves the efficacy of anticancer therapy. Clin Cancer Res 2008; 14(1): 270-80.
[http://dx.doi.org/10.1158/1078-0432.CCR-07-1562] [PMID: 18172279]

[2] Brown JM. Tumor microenvironment and the response to anticancer therapy. Cancer Biol Ther 2002; 1(5): 453-8.
[http://dx.doi.org/10.4161/cbt.1.5.157] [PMID: 12496469]

[3] Poluzzi C, Iozzo RV, Schaefer L. Endostatin and endorepellin: A common route of action for similar angiostatic cancer avengers. Adv Drug Deliv Rev 2016; 97: 156-73.
[http://dx.doi.org/10.1016/j.addr.2015.10.012] [PMID: 26518982]

[4] Trédan O, Galmarini CM, Patel K, Tannock IF. Drug resistance and the solid tumor microenvironment. J Natl Cancer Inst 2007; 99(19): 1441-54.
[http://dx.doi.org/10.1093/jnci/djm135] [PMID: 17895480]

[5] Song X. Targeting cancer associated fibroblasts for cancer immunotherapy. Cancer Cell Microenviron 2014; 1: 1-5.

[6] Hu M, Polyak K. Molecular characterisation of the tumour microenvironment in breast cancer. Eur J Cancer 2008; 44(18): 2760-5.
[http://dx.doi.org/10.1016/j.ejca.2008.09.038] [PMID: 19026532]

[7] Joyce JA. Therapeutic targeting of the tumor microenvironment. Cancer Cell 2005; 7(6): 513-20.
[http://dx.doi.org/10.1016/j.ccr.2005.05.024] [PMID: 15950901]

[8] Luo H, Tu G, Liu Z, Liu M. Cancer-associated fibroblasts: a multifaceted driver of breast cancer progression. Cancer Lett 2015; 361(2): 155-63.
[http://dx.doi.org/10.1016/j.canlet.2015.02.018] [PMID: 25700776]

[9] Yang JD, Nakamura I, Roberts LR. The tumor microenvironment in hepatocellular carcinoma: current status and therapeutic targets. Semin Cancer Biol 2011; 21(1): 35-43.
[http://dx.doi.org/10.1016/j.semcancer.2010.10.007] [PMID: 20946957]

[10] Sainio A, Järveläinen H. Extracellular matrix macromolecules: potential tools and targets in cancer gene therapy. Mol Cell Ther 2014; 2: 14.
[http://dx.doi.org/10.1186/2052-8426-2-14] [PMID: 26056582]

[11] Tsai M, Chang W, Huang M, Kuo P. Tumor microenvironment: A new treatment target for cancer. ISRN Biochem 2014; 1-8.
[http://dx.doi.org/10.1155/2014/351959]

[12] Bhome R, Al Saihati HA, Goh RW, *et al.* Translational aspects in targeting the stromal tumour microenvironment: from bench to bedside. New Horiz Transl Med 2016; 3(1): 9-21.
[http://dx.doi.org/10.1016/j.nhtm.2016.03.001] [PMID: 27275004]

[13] Hazlehurst LA, Landowski TH, Dalton WS. Role of the tumor microenvironment in mediating de novo resistance to drugs and physiological mediators of cell death. Oncogene 2003; 22(47): 7396-402. [http://dx.doi.org/10.1038/sj.onc.1206943] [PMID: 14576847]

[14] Morikawa K, Walker SM, Jessup JM, Fidler IJ. *In vivo* selection of highly metastatic cells from surgical specimens of different primary human colon carcinomas implanted into nude mice. Cancer Res 1988; 48(7): 1943-8. [PMID: 3349467]

[15] Morikawa K, Walker SM, Nakajima M, Pathak S, Jessup JM, Fidler IJ. Influence of organ environment on the growth, selection, and metastasis of human colon carcinoma cells in nude mice. Cancer Res 1988; 48(23): 6863-71. [PMID: 2846163]

[16] Nakajima M, Morikawa K, Fabra A, Bucana CD, Fidler IJ. Influence of organ environment on extracellular matrix degradative activity and metastasis of human colon carcinoma cells. J Natl Cancer Inst 1990; 82(24): 1890-8. [http://dx.doi.org/10.1093/jnci/82.24.1890] [PMID: 2174463]

[17] Rajantie I, Ilmonen M, Alminaite A, Ozerdem U, Alitalo K, Salven P. Adult bone marrow-derived cells recruited during angiogenesis comprise precursors for periendothelial vascular mural cells. Blood 2004; 104(7): 2084-6. [http://dx.doi.org/10.1182/blood-2004-01-0336] [PMID: 15191949]

[18] Kharaishvili G, Simkova D, Bouchalova K, Gachechiladze M, Narsia N, Bouchal J. The role of cancer-associated fibroblasts, solid stress and other microenvironmental factors in tumor progression and therapy resistance. Cancer Cell Int 2014; 14: 41-9. [http://dx.doi.org/10.1186/1475-2867-14-41] [PMID: 24883045]

[19] Turley SJ, Cremasco V, Astarita JL. Immunological hallmarks of stromal cells in the tumour microenvironment. Nat Rev Immunol 2015; 15(11): 669-82. [http://dx.doi.org/10.1038/nri3902] [PMID: 26471778]

[20] Zhou L, Yang K, Andl T, Wickett RR, Zhang Y. Perspective of targeting cancer-associated fibroblasts in melanoma. J Cancer 2015; 6(8): 717-26. [http://dx.doi.org/10.7150/jca.10865] [PMID: 26185533]

[21] Stacker SA, Williams SP, Karnezis T, Shayan R, Fox SB, Achen MG. Lymphangiogenesis and lymphatic vessel remodelling in cancer. Nat Rev Cancer 2014; 14(3): 159-72. [http://dx.doi.org/10.1038/nrc3677] [PMID: 24561443]

[22] Morin MJ. From oncogene to drug: development of small molecule tyrosine kinase inhibitors as anti-tumor and anti-angiogenic agents. Oncogene 2000; 19(56): 6574-83. [http://dx.doi.org/10.1038/sj.onc.1204102] [PMID: 11426642]

[23] Arias JL. Drug targeting strategies in cancer treatment: an overview. Mini Rev Med Chem 2011; 11(1): 1-17. [http://dx.doi.org/10.2174/138955711793564024] [PMID: 21235512]

[24] Bailar JC III, Gornik HL. Cancer undefeated. N Engl J Med 1997; 336(22): 1569-74. [http://dx.doi.org/10.1056/NEJM199705293362206] [PMID: 9164814]

[25] Gerber DE. Targeted therapies: a new generation of cancer treatments. Am Fam Physician 2008; 77(3): 311-9. [PMID: 18297955]

[26] Danhier F, Feron O, Préat V. To exploit the tumor microenvironment: Passive and active tumor targeting of nanocarriers for anti-cancer drug delivery. J Control Release 2010; 148(2): 135-46. [http://dx.doi.org/10.1016/j.jconrel.2010.08.027] [PMID: 20797419]

[27] Di Paolo A, Bocci G. Drug distribution in tumors: mechanisms, role in drug resistance, and methods for modification. Curr Oncol Rep 2007; 9(2): 109-14.

[http://dx.doi.org/10.1007/s11912-007-0006-3] [PMID: 17288875]

[28]   Cowan DS, Hicks KO, Wilson WR. Multicellular membranes as an *in vitro* model for extravascular diffusion in tumours. Br J Cancer Suppl 1996; 27: S28-31.
[PMID: 8763841]

[29]   Tannock IF, Lee CM, Tunggal JK, Cowan DS, Egorin MJ. Limited penetration of anticancer drugs through tumor tissue: a potential cause of resistance of solid tumors to chemotherapy. Clin Cancer Res 2002; 8(3): 878-84.
[PMID: 11895922]

[30]   Minchinton AI, Tannock IF. Drug penetration in solid tumours. Nat Rev Cancer 2006; 6(8): 583-92.
[http://dx.doi.org/10.1038/nrc1893] [PMID: 16862189]

[31]   Pillai G. Nanomedicines for cancer therapy: An update of FDA approved and those under various stages of development. SOJ Pharm Pharm Sci 2014; 1: 1-13.
[http://dx.doi.org/10.15226/2374-6866/1/1/00109]

[32]   Rani K. A review on targeted drug delivery: Its entire focus on advanced therapeutics and diagnostics. SJAMS 2014; 2: 328-31.

[33]   Miele E, Spinelli GP, Miele E, Tomao F, Tomao S. Albumin-bound formulation of paclitaxel (Abraxane ABI-007) in the treatment of breast cancer. Int J Nanomedicine 2009; 4: 99-105.
[PMID: 19516888]

[34]   Hamaguchi T, Matsumura Y, Suzuki M, *et al.* NK105, a paclitaxel-incorporating micellar nanoparticle formulation, can extend *in vivo* antitumour activity and reduce the neurotoxicity of paclitaxel. Br J Cancer 2005; 92(7): 1240-6.
[http://dx.doi.org/10.1038/sj.bjc.6602479] [PMID: 15785749]

[35]   Werner ME, Cummings ND, Sethi M, *et al.* Preclinical evaluation of Genexol-PM, a nanoparticle formulation of paclitaxel, as a novel radiosensitizer for the treatment of non-small cell lung cancer. Int J Radiat Oncol Biol Phys 2013; 86(3): 463-8.
[http://dx.doi.org/10.1016/j.ijrobp.2013.02.009] [PMID: 23708084]

[36]   Kim DW, Kim SY, Kim HK, *et al.* Multicenter phase II trial of Genexol-PM, a novel Cremophor-free, polymeric micelle formulation of paclitaxel, with cisplatin in patients with advanced non-small-cell lung cancer. Ann Oncol 2007; 18(12): 2009-14.
[http://dx.doi.org/10.1093/annonc/mdm374] [PMID: 17785767]

[37]   Barenholz Y. Doxil®the first FDA-approved nano-drug: lessons learned. J Control Release 2012; 160(2): 117-34.
[http://dx.doi.org/10.1016/j.jconrel.2012.03.020] [PMID: 22484195]

[38]   Safra T, Muggia F, Jeffers S, *et al.* Pegylated liposomal doxorubicin (doxil): reduced clinical cardiotoxicity in patients reaching or exceeding cumulative doses of 500 mg/m2. Ann Oncol 2000; 11(8): 1029-33.
[http://dx.doi.org/10.1023/A:1008365716693] [PMID: 11038041]

[39]   Sarris AH, Hagemeister F, Romaguera J, *et al.* Liposomal vincristine in relapsed non-Hodgkins lymphomas: early results of an ongoing phase II trial. Ann Oncol 2000; 11(1): 69-72.
[http://dx.doi.org/10.1023/A:1008348010437] [PMID: 10690390]

[40]   Fassas A, Anagnostopoulos A. The use of liposomal daunorubicin (DaunoXome) in acute myeloid leukemia. Leuk Lymphoma 2005; 46(6): 795-802.
[http://dx.doi.org/10.1080/10428190500052438] [PMID: 16019523]

[41]   Gujral TS, Peshkin L, Kirschner MW. Exploiting polypharmacology for drug target deconvolution. Proc Natl Acad Sci USA 2014; 111(13): 5048-53.
[http://dx.doi.org/10.1073/pnas.1403080111] [PMID: 24707051]

[42]   Gramoun A, Shorey S, Bashutski JD, *et al.* Effects of Vitaxin, a novel therapeutic in trial for metastatic bone tumors, on osteoclast functions *in vitro*. J Cell Biochem 2007; 102(2): 341-52.

[http://dx.doi.org/10.1002/jcb.21296] [PMID: 17390341]

[43]　Stupp R, Hegi ME, Gorlia T, *et al.* European Organisation for Research and Treatment of Cancer (EORTC); Canadian Brain Tumor Consortium; CENTRIC study team. Cilengitide combined with standard treatment for patients with newly diagnosed glioblastoma with methylated MGMT promoter (CENTRIC EORTC 2607122072 study): a multicentre, randomised, open-label, phase 3 trial. Lancet Oncol 2014; 15(10): 1100-8.
[http://dx.doi.org/10.1016/S1470-2045(14)70379-1] [PMID: 25163906]

[44]　Vu T, Sliwkowski MX, Claret FX. Personalized drug combinations to overcome trastuzumab resistance in HER2-positive breast cancer. BBA-Rev Cancer 2014; 1846: 353-65.

[45]　Burotto M, Manasanch EE, Wilkerson J, Fojo T. Gefitinib and erlotinib in metastatic non-small cell lung cancer: a meta-analysis of toxicity and efficacy of randomized clinical trials. Oncologist 2015; 20(4): 400-10.
[http://dx.doi.org/10.1634/theoncologist.2014-0154] [PMID: 25795635]

[46]　Kollmannsberger C, Soulieres D, Wong R, Scalera A, Gaspo R, Bjarnason G. Sunitinib therapy for metastatic renal cell carcinoma: recommendations for management of side effects. Can Urol Assoc J 2007; 1(2) (Suppl.): S41-54.
[PMID: 18542784]

[47]　Mas-Moruno C, Rechenmacher F, Kessler H. Cilengitide: the first anti-angiogenic small molecule drug candidate design, synthesis and clinical evaluation. Anticancer Agents Med Chem 2010; 10(10): 753-68.
[http://dx.doi.org/10.2174/187152010794728639] [PMID: 21269250]

[48]　Hu Q, Sun W, Lu Y, *et al.* Tumor microenvironment-mediated constraction and deconstraction of extracellular drug-delivery depots. Nano Lett 2016; 16(2): 1118-26.
[http://dx.doi.org/10.1021/acs.nanolett.5b04343] [PMID: 26785163]

[49]　Pepper MS. Manipulating angiogenesis. From basic science to the bedside. Arterioscler Thromb Vasc Biol 1997; 17(4): 605-19.
[http://dx.doi.org/10.1161/01.ATV.17.4.605] [PMID: 9108772]

[50]　Carmeliet P. Angiogenesis in health and disease. Nat Med 2003; 9(6): 653-60.
[http://dx.doi.org/10.1038/nm0603-653] [PMID: 12778163]

[51]　Hanahan D, Folkman J. Patterns and emerging mechanisms of the angiogenic switch during tumorigenesis. Cell 1996; 86(3): 353-64.
[http://dx.doi.org/10.1016/S0092-8674(00)80108-7] [PMID: 8756718]

[52]　Folkman J. Angiogenesis and apoptosis. Semin Cancer Biol 2003; 13(2): 159-67.
[http://dx.doi.org/10.1016/S1044-579X(02)00133-5] [PMID: 12654259]

[53]　El-Kenawi AE, El-Remessy AB. Angiogenesis inhibitors in cancer therapy: mechanistic perspective on classification and treatment rationales. Br J Pharmacol 2013; 170(4): 712-29.
[http://dx.doi.org/10.1111/bph.12344] [PMID: 23962094]

[54]　Jain RK. Normalizing tumor vasculature with anti-angiogenic therapy: a new paradigm for combination therapy. Nat Med 2001; 7(9): 987-9.
[http://dx.doi.org/10.1038/nm0901-987] [PMID: 11533692]

[55]　Durand RE, Olive PL. Resistance of tumor cells to chemo- and radiotherapy modulated by the three-dimensional architecture of solid tumors and spheroids. Methods Cell Biol 2001; 64: 211-33.
[http://dx.doi.org/10.1016/S0091-679X(01)64015-9] [PMID: 11070841]

[56]　Jain RK. Determinants of tumor blood flow: a review. Cancer Res 1988; 48(10): 2641-58.
[PMID: 3282647]

[57]　Carmeliet P, Jain RK. Angiogenesis in cancer and other diseases. Nature 2000; 407(6801): 249-57.
[http://dx.doi.org/10.1038/35025220] [PMID: 11001068]

[58]   Yonenaga Y, Mori A, Onodera H, *et al.* Absence of smooth muscle actin-positive pericyte coverage of tumor vessels correlates with hematogenous metastasis and prognosis of colorectal cancer patients. Oncology 2005; 69(2): 159-66.
[http://dx.doi.org/10.1159/000087840] [PMID: 16127287]

[59]   Hashizume H, Baluk P, Morikawa S, *et al.* Openings between defective endothelial cells explain tumor vessel leakiness. Am J Pathol 2000; 156(4): 1363-80.
[http://dx.doi.org/10.1016/S0002-9440(10)65006-7] [PMID: 10751361]

[60]   Heldin CH, Rubin K, Pietras K, Ostman A. High interstitial fluid pressure - an obstacle in cancer therapy. Nat Rev Cancer 2004; 4(10): 806-13.
[http://dx.doi.org/10.1038/nrc1456] [PMID: 15510161]

[61]   Boucher Y, Baxter LT, Jain RK. Interstitial pressure gradients in tissue-isolated and subcutaneous tumors: implications for therapy. Cancer Res 1990; 50(15): 4478-84.
[PMID: 2369726]

[62]   Jain RK. Normalization of tumor vasculature: an emerging concept in antiangiogenic therapy. Science 2005; 307(5706): 58-62.
[http://dx.doi.org/10.1126/science.1104819] [PMID: 15637262]

[63]   Tong RT, Boucher Y, Kozin SV, Winkler F, Hicklin DJ, Jain RK. Vascular normalization by vascular endothelial growth factor receptor 2 blockade induces a pressure gradient across the vasculature and improves drug penetration in tumors. Cancer Res 2004; 64(11): 3731-6.
[http://dx.doi.org/10.1158/0008-5472.CAN-04-0074] [PMID: 15172975]

[64]   Cook KM, Figg WD. Angiogenesis inhibitors: current strategies and future prospects. CA Cancer J Clin 2010; 60(4): 222-43.
[http://dx.doi.org/10.3322/caac.20075] [PMID: 20554717]

[65]   Kerbel RS. Inhibition of tumor angiogenesis as a strategy to circumvent acquired resistance to anti-cancer therapeutic agents. BioEssays 1991; 13(1): 31-6.
[http://dx.doi.org/10.1002/bies.950130106] [PMID: 1722975]

[66]   Mabeta P, Pepper MS. A comparative study on the anti-angiogenic effects of DNA-damaging and cytoskeletal-disrupting agents. Angiogenesis 2009; 12(1): 81-90.
[http://dx.doi.org/10.1007/s10456-009-9134-8] [PMID: 19214765]

[67]   Mabeta P, Pepper MS. Inhibition of hemangioma development in a syngeneic mouse model correlates with bcl-2 suppression and the inhibition of Akt kinase activity. Angiogenesis 2012; 15(1): 131-9.
[http://dx.doi.org/10.1007/s10456-011-9248-7] [PMID: 22198238]

[68]   Grothey A, Sugrue MM, Purdie DM, *et al.* Bevacizumab beyond first progression is associated with prolonged overall survival in metastatic colorectal cancer: results from a large observational cohort study (BRiTE). J Clin Oncol 2008; 26(33): 5326-34.
[http://dx.doi.org/10.1200/JCO.2008.16.3212] [PMID: 18854571]

[69]   Papadopoulos N, Martin J, Ruan Q, *et al.* Binding and neutralization of vascular endothelial growth factor (VEGF) and related ligands by VEGF Trap, ranibizumab and bevacizumab. Angiogenesis 2012; 15(2): 171-85.
[http://dx.doi.org/10.1007/s10456-011-9249-6] [PMID: 22302382]

[70]   Ferrara N, Hillan KJ, Gerber HP, Novotny W. Discovery and development of bevacizumab, an anti-VEGF antibody for treating cancer. Nat Rev Drug Discov 2004; 3(5): 391-400.
[http://dx.doi.org/10.1038/nrd1381] [PMID: 15136787]

[71]   Bennouna J, Sastre J, Arnold D, *et al.* ML18147 Study Investigators. Continuation of bevacizumab after first progression in metastatic colorectal cancer (ML18147): a randomised phase 3 trial. Lancet Oncol 2013; 14(1): 29-37.
[http://dx.doi.org/10.1016/S1470-2045(12)70477-1] [PMID: 23168366]

[72]   Ng EW, Shima DT, Calias P, Cunningham ET Jr, Guyer DR, Adamis AP. Pegaptanib, a targeted anti-

VEGF aptamer for ocular vascular disease. Nat Rev Drug Discov 2006; 5(2): 123-32.
[http://dx.doi.org/10.1038/nrd1955] [PMID: 16518379]

[73]   Bhise NS, Shmueli RB, Sunshine JC, Tzeng SY, Green JJ. Drug delivery strategies for therapeutic angiogenesis and antiangiogenesis. Expert Opin Drug Deliv 2011; 8(4): 485-504.
[http://dx.doi.org/10.1517/17425247.2011.558082] [PMID: 21338327]

[74]   Zhang X, Yang XR, Huang XW, *et al.* Sorafenib in treatment of patients with advanced hepatocellular carcinoma: a systematic review. HBPD INT 2012; 11(5): 458-66.
[http://dx.doi.org/10.1016/S1499-3872(12)60209-4] [PMID: 23060390]

[75]   Griffioen AW, Mans LA, de Graaf AM, *et al.* Rapid angiogenesis onset after discontinuation of sunitinib treatment of renal cell carcinoma patients. Clin Cancer Res 2012; 18(14): 3961-71.
[http://dx.doi.org/10.1158/1078-0432.CCR-12-0002] [PMID: 22573349]

[76]   Mankal P, OReilly E. Sunitinib malate for the treatment of pancreas malignancieswhere does it fit? Expert Opin Pharmacother 2013; 14(6): 783-92.
[http://dx.doi.org/10.1517/14656566.2013.776540] [PMID: 23458511]

[77]   van Cruijsen H, Voest EE, Punt CJ, *et al.* Phase I evaluation of cediranib, a selective VEGFR signalling inhibitor, in combination with gefitinib in patients with advanced tumours. Eur J Cancer 2010; 46(5): 901-11.
[http://dx.doi.org/10.1016/j.ejca.2009.12.023] [PMID: 20061136]

[78]   Pietras K, Rubin K, Sjöblom T, *et al.* Inhibition of PDGF receptor signaling in tumor stroma enhances antitumor effect of chemotherapy. Cancer Res 2002; 62(19): 5476-84.
[PMID: 12359756]

[79]   Pietras K, Sjöblom T, Rubin K, Heldin CH, Ostman A. PDGF receptors as cancer drug targets. Cancer Cell 2003; 3(5): 439-43.
[http://dx.doi.org/10.1016/S1535-6108(03)00089-8] [PMID: 12781361]

[80]   Pepper MS. Role of the matrix metalloproteinase and plasminogen activator-plasmin systems in angiogenesis. Arterioscler Thromb Vasc Biol 2001; 21(7): 1104-17.
[http://dx.doi.org/10.1161/hq0701.093685] [PMID: 11451738]

[81]   Damiano JS, Cress AE, Hazlehurst LA, Shtil AA, Dalton WS. Cell adhesion mediated drug resistance (CAM-DR): role of integrins and resistance to apoptosis in human myeloma cell lines. Blood 1999; 93(5): 1658-67.
[PMID: 10029595]

[82]   Weaver VM, Lelièvre S, Lakins JN, *et al.* beta4 integrin-dependent formation of polarized three-dimensional architecture confers resistance to apoptosis in normal and malignant mammary epithelium. Cancer Cell 2002; 2(3): 205-16.
[http://dx.doi.org/10.1016/S1535-6108(02)00125-3] [PMID: 12242153]

[83]   Besse B, Tsao LC, Chao DT, *et al.* Phase Ib safety and pharmacokinetic study of volociximab, an anti-α5β1 integrin antibody, in combination with carboplatin and paclitaxel in advanced non-small-cell lung cancer. Ann Oncol 2013; 24(1): 90-6.
[http://dx.doi.org/10.1093/annonc/mds281] [PMID: 22904239]

[84]   Almokadem S, Belani CP. Volociximab in cancer. Expert Opin Biol Ther 2012; 12(2): 251-7.
[http://dx.doi.org/10.1517/14712598.2012.646985] [PMID: 22192080]

[85]   Cameron D, Brown J, Dent R, Jackisch C, Mackey J, Pivot X, *et al.* Primary results of BEATRICE, a randomized phaseIII trial evaluating adjuvent bevacizumab-containing therapy in triple-negative breast cancer. Cancer Res 2012; •••: 72.

[86]   Robert NJ, Diéras V, Glaspy J, *et al.* RIBBON-1: randomized, double-blind, placebo-controlled, phase III trial of chemotherapy with or without bevacizumab for first-line treatment of human epidermal growth factor receptor 2-negative, locally recurrent or metastatic breast cancer. J Clin Oncol 2011; 29(10): 1252-60.

[http://dx.doi.org/10.1200/JCO.2010.28.0982] [PMID: 21383283]

[87]   Brufsky AM, Hurvitz S, Perez E, *et al.* RIBBON-2: a randomized, double-blind, placebo-controlled, phase III trial evaluating the efficacy and safety of bevacizumab in combination with chemotherapy for second-line treatment of human epidermal growth factor receptor 2-negative metastatic breast cancer. J Clin Oncol 2011; 29(32): 4286-93.
[http://dx.doi.org/10.1200/JCO.2010.34.1255] [PMID: 21990397]

[88]   Miles DW, Chan A, Dirix LY, *et al.* Phase III study of bevacizumab plus docetaxel compared with placebo plus docetaxel for the first-line treatment of human epidermal growth factor receptor 2-negative metastatic breast cancer. J Clin Oncol 2010; 28(20): 3239-47.
[http://dx.doi.org/10.1200/JCO.2008.21.6457] [PMID: 20498403]

[89]   Mancuso MR, Davis R, Norberg SM, *et al.* Rapid vascular regrowth in tumors after reversal of VEGF inhibition. J Clin Invest 2006; 116(10): 2610-21.
[http://dx.doi.org/10.1172/JCI24612] [PMID: 17016557]

[90]   Wolter P, Beuselinck B, Pans S, Schöffski P. Flare-up: an often unreported phenomenon nevertheless familiar to oncologists prescribing tyrosine kinase inhibitors. Acta Oncol 2009; 48(4): 621-4.
[http://dx.doi.org/10.1080/02841860802609574] [PMID: 19107622]

[91]   Desar IM, Mulder SF, Stillebroer AB, *et al.* The reverse side of the victory: flare up of symptoms after discontinuation of sunitinib or sorafenib in renal cell cancer patients. A report of three cases. Acta Oncol 2009; 48(6): 927-31.
[http://dx.doi.org/10.1080/02841860902974167] [PMID: 19452305]

[92]   Van Cutsem E, Tabernero J, Lakomy R, *et al.* Addition of aflibercept to fluorouracil, leucovorin, and irinotecan improves survival in a phase III randomized trial in patients with metastatic colorectal cancer previously treated with an oxaliplatin-based regimen. J Clin Oncol 2012; 30(28): 3499-506.
[http://dx.doi.org/10.1200/JCO.2012.42.8201] [PMID: 22949147]

[93]   Pietrantonio F, Perrone F, Biondani P, *et al.* Single agent panitumumab in KRAS wild-type metastatic colorectal cancer patients following cetuximab-based regimens: Clinical outcome and biomarkers of efficacy. Cancer Biol Ther 2013; 14(12): 1098-103.
[http://dx.doi.org/10.4161/cbt.26343] [PMID: 24025413]

[94]   McCormack PL, Keam SJ. Spotlight on bevacizumab in metastatic colorectal cancer. BioDrugs 2008; 22(5): 339-41.
[http://dx.doi.org/10.2165/00063030-200822050-00006] [PMID: 18778115]

[95]   Delea TE, Amdahl J, Chit A, Amonkar MM. Cost-effectiveness of lapatinib plus letrozole in her2-positive, hormone receptor-positive metastatic breast cancer in Canada. Curr Oncol 2013; 20(5): e371-87.
[http://dx.doi.org/10.3747/co.20.1394] [PMID: 24155635]

[96]   Alitalo A, Detmar M. Interaction of tumor cells and lymphatic vessels in cancer progression. Oncogene 2012; 31(42): 4499-508.
[http://dx.doi.org/10.1038/onc.2011.602] [PMID: 22179834]

[97]   Caunt M, Mak J, Liang WC, *et al.* Blocking neuropilin-2 function inhibits tumor cell metastasis. Cancer Cell 2008; 13(4): 331-42.
[http://dx.doi.org/10.1016/j.ccr.2008.01.029] [PMID: 18394556]

[98]   Lin J, Lalani AS, Harding TC, *et al.* Inhibition of lymphogenous metastasis using adeno-associated virus-mediated gene transfer of a soluble VEGFR-3 decoy receptor. Cancer Res 2005; 65(15): 6901-9.
[http://dx.doi.org/10.1158/0008-5472.CAN-05-0408] [PMID: 16061674]

[99]   He Y, Kozaki K, Karpanen T, *et al.* Suppression of tumor lymphangiogenesis and lymph node metastasis by blocking vascular endothelial growth factor receptor 3 signaling. J Natl Cancer Inst 2002; 94(11): 819-25.
[http://dx.doi.org/10.1093/jnci/94.11.819] [PMID: 12048269]

[100] García-Caballero M, Blacher S, Paupert J, Quesada AR, Medina MA, Noël A. Novel application assigned to toluquinol: inhibition of lymphangiogenesis by interfering with VEGF-C/VEGFR-3 signalling pathway. Br J Pharmacol 2016; 173(12): 1966-87.
[http://dx.doi.org/10.1111/bph.13488] [PMID: 27018653]

[101] Xu Y, Lin H, Meng N, *et al.* YL529, a novel, orally available multikinase inhibitor, potently inhibits angiogenesis and tumour growth in preclinical models. Br J Pharmacol 2013; 169(8): 1766-80.
[http://dx.doi.org/10.1111/bph.12216] [PMID: 23594209]

[102] Au JL, Yeung BZ, Wientjes MG, Lu Z, Wientjes MG. Delivery of cancer therapeutics to extracellular and intracellular targets: Determinants, barriers, challenges and opportunities. Adv Drug Deliv Rev 2016; 97: 280-301.
[http://dx.doi.org/10.1016/j.addr.2015.12.002] [PMID: 26686425]

[103] Wong GS, Rustgi AK. Matricellular proteins: priming the tumour microenvironment for cancer development and metastasis. Br J Cancer 2013; 108(4): 755-61.
[http://dx.doi.org/10.1038/bjc.2012.592] [PMID: 23322204]

[104] Deryugina EI, Quigley JP. Tumor angiogenesis: MMP-mediated induction of intravasation- and metastasis-sustaining neovasculature. Matrix Biol 2015; 44-46: 94-112.
[http://dx.doi.org/10.1016/j.matbio.2015.04.004] [PMID: 25912949]

[105] Murphy-Ullrich JE, Sage EH. Revisiting the matricellular concept. Matrix Biol 2014; 37: 1-14.
[http://dx.doi.org/10.1016/j.matbio.2014.07.005] [PMID: 25064829]

[106] Jun JI, Lau LF. Taking aim at the extracellular matrix: CCN proteins as emerging therapeutic targets. Nat Rev Drug Discov 2011; 10(12): 945-63.
[http://dx.doi.org/10.1038/nrd3599] [PMID: 22129992]

[107] Schaefer L, Reinhardt DP. Special issue: Extracellular matrix: Therapeutic tools and targets in cancer treatment. Adv Drug Deliv Rev 2016; 97: 1-3.
[http://dx.doi.org/10.1016/j.addr.2016.01.001] [PMID: 26872878]

[108] Jain RK, Stylianopoulos T. Delivering nanomedicine to solid tumors. Nat Rev Clin Oncol 2010; 7(11): 653-64.
[http://dx.doi.org/10.1038/nrclinonc.2010.139] [PMID: 20838415]

[109] Goodman SL, Picard M. Integrins as therapeutic targets. Trends Pharmacol Sci 2012; 33(7): 405-12.
[http://dx.doi.org/10.1016/j.tips.2012.04.002] [PMID: 22633092]

[110] Magzoub M, Jin S, Verkman AS. Enhanced macromolecule diffusion deep in tumors after enzymatic digestion of extracellular matrix collagen and its associated proteoglycan decorin. FASEB J 2008; 22(1): 276-84.
[http://dx.doi.org/10.1096/fj.07-9150com] [PMID: 17761521]

[111] Feng Q, Zhang Z, Shea MJ, *et al.* An epigenomic approach to therapy for tamoxifen-resistant breast cancer. Cell Res 2014; 24(7): 809-19.
[http://dx.doi.org/10.1038/cr.2014.71] [PMID: 24874954]

[112] Kalluri R, Zeisberg M. Fibroblasts in cancer. Nat Rev Cancer 2006; 6(5): 392-401.
[http://dx.doi.org/10.1038/nrc1877] [PMID: 16572188]

[113] Frantz C, Stewart KM, Weaver VM. The extracellular matrix at a glance. J Cell Sci 2010; 123(Pt 24): 4195-200.
[http://dx.doi.org/10.1242/jcs.023820] [PMID: 21123617]

[114] Kidd S, Spaeth E, Watson K, *et al.* Origins of the tumor microenvironment: quantitative assessment of adipose-derived and bone marrow-derived stroma. PLoS One 2012; 7(2): e30563.
[http://dx.doi.org/10.1371/journal.pone.0030563] [PMID: 22363446]

[115] Schäffler A, Büchler C. Concise review: adipose tissue-derived stromal cellsbasic and clinical implications for novel cell-based therapies. Stem Cells 2007; 25(4): 818-27.

[http://dx.doi.org/10.1634/stemcells.2006-0589] [PMID: 17420225]

[116] Landskron G, De la Fuente M, Thuwajit P, Thuwajit C, Hermoso MA. Chronic inflammation and cytokines in the tumor microenvironment. J Immunol Res 2014; 1-19.

[117] Chang AI, Schwertschkow AH, Nolta JA, Wu J. Involvement of mesenchymal stem cells in cancer progression and metastases. Curr Cancer Drug Targets 2015; 15(2): 88-98.
[http://dx.doi.org/10.2174/1568009615666150126154151] [PMID: 25619387]

[118] Song X-T. Targeting cancer associated fibroblasts for cancer immunotherapy. Cancer Cell Microenviron 2014; 1: 1-5.

[119] Coussens LM, Werb Z. Inflammation and cancer. Nature 2002; 420(6917): 860-7.
[http://dx.doi.org/10.1038/nature01322] [PMID: 12490959]

[120] Colotta F, Allavena P, Sica A, Garlanda C, Mantovani A. Cancer-related inflammation, the seventh hallmark of cancer: links to genetic instability. Carcinogenesis 2009; 30(7): 1073-81.
[http://dx.doi.org/10.1093/carcin/bgp127] [PMID: 19468060]

[121] Hanahan D, Coussens LM. Accessories to the crime: functions of cells recruited to the tumor microenvironment. Cancer Cell 2012; 21(3): 309-22.
[http://dx.doi.org/10.1016/j.ccr.2012.02.022] [PMID: 22439926]

[122] Williams CB, Yeh ES, Soloff AC. Tumor-associated macrophages: unwitting accomplices in breast cancer malignancy. NPJ Breast Cancer 2016; 2: 1-12.
[http://dx.doi.org/10.1038/npjbcancer.2015.25] [PMID: 26998515]

[123] Pradel LP, Ooi CH, Romagnoli S, *et al.* Macrophage susceptibility to emactuzumab (RG7155) treatment. Mol Cancer Ther 2016. molcanther-0157.

[124] Weber JS, ODay S, Urba W, *et al.* Phase I/II study of ipilimumab for patients with metastatic melanoma. J Clin Oncol 2008; 26(36): 5950-6.
[http://dx.doi.org/10.1200/JCO.2008.16.1927] [PMID: 19018089]

[125] Pienta KJ, Machiels JP, Schrijvers D, *et al.* Phase 2 study of carlumab (CNTO 888), a human monoclonal antibody against CC-chemokine ligand 2 (CCL2), in metastatic castration-resistant prostate cancer. Invest New Drugs 2013; 31(3): 760-8.

[126] Daquinag AC, Tseng C, Zhang Y, *et al.* Targeted proapoptotic peptides depleting adipose stromal cells inhibit tumor growth. Mol Ther 2016; 24(1): 34-40.
[http://dx.doi.org/10.1038/mt.2015.155] [PMID: 26316391]

[127] Zhang Y, Daquinag AC, Amaya-Manzanares F, Sirin O, Tseng C, Kolonin MG. Stromal progenitor cells from endogenous adipose tissue contribute to pericytes and adipocytes that populate the tumor microenvironment. Cancer Res 2012; 72(20): 5198-208.
[http://dx.doi.org/10.1158/0008-5472.CAN-12-0294] [PMID: 23071132]

CHAPTER 4

Current and Emerging Cancer Therapies for Treatment of Hepatocellular Carcinoma

Sarwat Fatima[1,2,*]**, Nikki P. Lee**[3] **and Zhao Xiang Bian**[1,2]

[1] *Lab of Brain and Gut Research, Centre of Clinical Research for Chinese Medicine, School of Chinese Medicine, Hong Kong Baptist University, Kowloon Tong, Hong Kong SAR, China*

[2] *Centre for Cancer and Inflammation Research, School of Chinese Medicine, Hong Kong Baptist University, Kowloon Tong, Hong Kong SAR, China*

[3] *Department of Surgery, The University of Hong Kong, Pokfulam, Hong Kong SAR, China*

Abstract: Hepatocellular carcinoma (HCC) is one of the leading causes of cancer related deaths worldwide, especially in Asia. Late diagnosis and/or underlying cirrhosis, and limited treatment options with marginal clinical benefit are the reasons for its dismal prognosis. Surgical resection and liver transplantation are curative treatment options but are suitable for patients with small tumours or well-compensated liver diseases. For patients with non-resectable HCC, treatment options include ablative and systemic therapies. However, the results are unsatisfactory with limited long-term survival. In the last few years there has been active research in the area of molecularly targeted agents for HCC including anti-angiogenic therapy, immunotherapy, antiviral therapy, and other agents targeting mammalian target of rapamycin (mTOR), and c-met among others. This chapter will look into current treatment options, discuss their advantages and disadvantages, as well as introduce new therapies that are under clinical investigation but not yet recommended by acceptable guidelines. Although there is tremendous research in progress, the treatment modalities offer limited survival benefit and thus the battle against HCC is far from over.

Keywords: Anti-angiogenic therapy, Antiviral therapy, Chemotherapy, c-Met inhibitors, Hepatocellular carcinoma, Immune based therapy, Local ablative therapy, mTOR inhibitors, Sorafenib, TACE.

INTRODUCTION

Liver cancer is the second leading cause of cancer-related deaths worldwide. In 2012, there were 782,000 new cases and an estimated 746,000 deaths [1]. Among

* **Corresponding author Sarwat Fatima:** Lab of Brain and Gut Research, Centre of Clinical Research for Chinese Medicine, and Centre for Cancer and Inflammation Research, School of Chinese Medicine, Hong Kong Baptist University, Kowloon Tong, Hong Kong SAR, China; Tel: (+852) 34112072; Fax: (+852) 34112929; E-mail: sarwat@hkbu.edu.hk, nikkilee@hku.hk

Atta-ur-Rahman & M. Iqbal Choudhary (Eds.)

primary liver cancers, HCC is the most common subtype. The highest rates of HCC are reported in south-east Asia with more than 50% of HCC cases occurring in China. The incidence of HCC is also on the rise in the western world due to an increase in hepatitis C virus (HCV) infection [2].

The main aetiology of HCC is underlying cirrhosis with about 80%-90% of patients with cirrhosis go on to develop HCC and the remaining 10%-20% develop HCC without cirrhosis. Cirrhosis is caused by chronic hepatitis B virus (HBV) or HCV infection, fatty liver diseases, exposure to aflatoxins, chronic alcohol intake, non-alcoholic steatohepatitis (NASH) or less commonly due to other factors such as autoimmune or genetic metabolic liver diseases (hereditary hemochromatosis, α1-antitrypsin deficiency) [3, 4].

HCC suffers from a high rate of mortality due to lack of diagnostic methods and limited treatment options for patients with advanced HCC. Despite efforts to screen for early HCC by ultrasound screening and serum alpha fetoprotein (AFP) levels, patients are commonly asymptomatic until decompensation of their cirrhosis resulting from replacement of functional liver tissue by tumour tissue. Ultrasound surveillance is operator-dependant with low reproducibility and AFP levels are also dysregulated in benign liver diseases [5]. Furthermore, about 15% of patients show metastasis at the time of diagnosis. The most common sites for metastasis are the lungs, abdominal lymph nodes, bone, and adrenal glands [6]. The American Association for the Study of Liver Diseases (AASLD) and the European Association for the Study of the Liver (EASL) both endorse the Barcelona clinic liver cancer (BCLC) staging classification as criteria for the management of patients with HCC. Table **1** lists the BCLC classification. Treatment options for HCC are stage dependent and can be categorised into three groups: curative, palliative and symptomatic (Fig. **1**). For early stage tumours, curative treatment options include resection and percutaneous ablation which may achieve a five year survival rate of 70%. Patients who are not suitable for first-line therapy are treated with the next BCLC stage. This includes HCC patients with no macrovascular invasion or extrahepatic spread. These patients are suitable for transarterial chemoembolization (TACE). However, patients with advanced-stage HCC, with evidence of portal invasion, lymph node involvement and distant metastasis have 1 year survival rate of only 50% and before the introduction of sorafenib there was no treatment option shown to improve survival [7]. This book chapter aims to review the current and emerging treatment modalities for HCC patients.

Table 1. BCLC staging classification of HCC [8, 9].

Stage	PST	Tumour Characteristics		Liver Function
		Tumour Stage	Okuda Stage	
Stage A (early HCC)				
A1	0	Single tumour, <5cm	I	No portal hypertension and normal bilirubin
A2	0	Single tumour, <5cm	I	Portal hypertension and normal bilirubin
A3	0	Single tumour, <5cm	I	Portal hypertension and abnormal bilirubin
A4	0	3 tumours < 3cm each	I-II	Child-pugh A-B
Stage B (intermediate HCC)	0	Large multinodular	I-II	Child-pugh A-B
Stage C (advanced HCC)	1-2[a]	Portal invasion, nodal metastases, distant metastases	I-II	Child-pugh A-B
Stage D (end stage-HCC)	3-4[b]	Any	III[b]	Child-pugh C[b]

PST: Performance status test; Stage A and B, all criteria should to be fulfilled; [a]: Stage C, at least one criteria to be fulfilled, PST 1-2 or portal invasion/extrahepatic spread; [b]: Stage D, at least one criteria to be fulfilled, PST 3-4 or Okuda stage III/ Child-pugh C.

Surgical and Local Ablative Therapies

Surgery is the preferred treatment option for HCC patients because it is associated with a 5-year survival rate of 70% [7]. However, at the time of diagnosis, only about 10%-30% of HCC patients are amenable to liver resection. According to the BCLC guideline, surgery is limited to only early stage cancers (a single HCC < 5cm in diameter or up to 3 HCCs < 3cm in diameter) with good hepatic function and performance status. This criteria is sometimes considered restrictive as tumour size and number are not considered contraindication for surgery as long as there is sufficient hepatic reserve and that the tumour is resectable [10]. Studies have shown that resection may be the only hope for cure in large multinodular HCC with 5-year overall survival (OS) and disease-free survival of 39% and 26% respectively being achievable [11, 12]. For patients without cirrhosis, the least remnant liver volume for surgical resection is about 25% and 50% for HCC patients with cirrhosis [12].

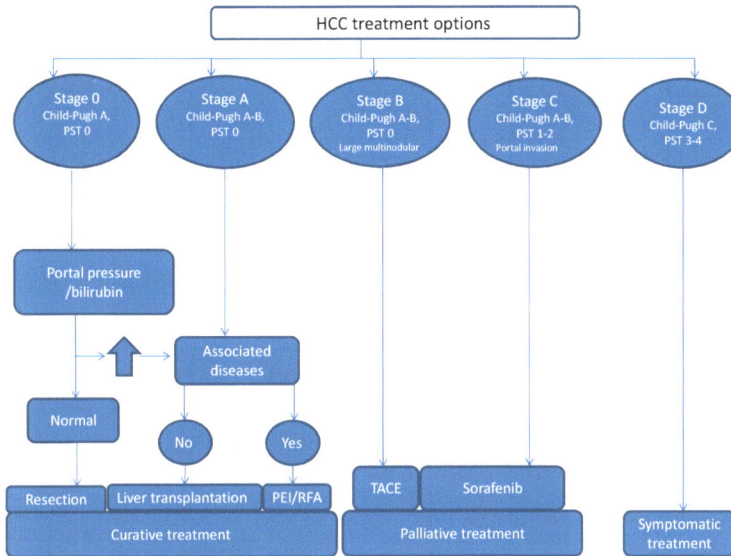

Fig. (1). The BCLC classification system links the treatment options for HCC. PEI: percutaneous ethanol; RFA: radio frequency ablation; TACE; transarterial chemoembolization.

An important factor post-surgery is the high risk of recurrence. Five-year recurrence rate of up to 68% has been reported after liver resection in early-stage HCC. Several factors including elevated AFP levels, presence of satellite nodules, cirrhosis, and HBV surface antigens have been found to be associated to tumour recurrence [13, 14].

A more sophisticated surgical procedure called laparoscopic resection has been reported to be associated to reduce operative and postoperative morbidities. Several studies have reported that laparoscopic hepatectomy results in decreased blood loss, fewer postoperative complications, shorter hospital stay with no difference in recurrence or survival rates [15, 16]. However, these studies should be interpreted with caution as they are retrospective studies with no randomised controlled trials.

Liver Transplantation (LTx)

LTx is the preferred treatment option for HCC patients with decompensated cirrhosis as LTx not only removes primary tumour but it also treats the underlying tumour-generating cirrhosis. The Milan criteria is a benchmark used to select patients with cirrhosis and HCC for LTx. It is recommended to HCC patients with tumours within the Milan criteria (a single lesion ≥5cm, or up to three lesions ≤3cm each) yielding a 5-year OS rate of 75% and patients whose tumours were outside the Milan criteria had poorer outcomes [17]. Recently, Vitale A *et al.* [18] reported that the BCLC staging could also be used to predict prognosis of HCC patients waiting for LTx. Enhanced survival benefit was observed for patients with advanced liver cirrhosis (BCLC stage D) and in those with intermediate tumours (BCLC stages B-C), regardless of the Milan criteria as long as there is absence of macroscopic vascular invasion and extra-hepatic disease. A median 5-year transplant benefit of 11.19 months for BCLC 0, 13.49 months for BCLC A, 17.36 months for BCLC B-C, and 28.46 months for BCLC D was reported. Thus, the BCLC system could potentially improve the selection process for LTx.

The major limitations of LTx are organ shortage and the long waiting time for transplantation. In the context of organ shortage, HCC patients also have to compete with non-cancer patients for transplants. Thus, to limit transplantation to patients whose outcomes are comparable to those who do not have HCC, a strict criteria is used, as mentioned above. Although LTx has good survival outcomes the long wait for a donor organ leads to dropout due to disease progression. While patients are waiting for LTx their tumours may progress and develop distant metastases and this may lead to patients losing their candidacy for LTx. Other complications include rejection and complications from immunosuppression may affect long term survival of transplant recipients [19].

Several factors are considered before deciding between surgical resection and LTx. Early-stage HCC patients with insufficient hepatic reserve for surgical resection would undergo LTx as the only treatment option. However, patients with large HCC but with adequate hepatic function would undergo surgical resection. In the case of HCC patients with early-stage HCC and well compensated cirrhosis, the choice between surgical resection and LTx would depend on the availability of donor organ and the LTx waiting list dropout rate resulting from disease progression [20]. In 2012, Rahman A *et al.* [21] performed a systematic review comparing the survival rates and recurrence rates of surgical resection and LTx. The 5-year OS rate ranged from 40% to 70% for resection and from 52% to 81% for LTx, suggesting no significant difference in survival between the two treatment options. Another meta-analysis by Dhir M *et al.* [22] also found no difference in survival outcomes of the two groups. In 2015, Kaido T *et al.* [23] recently compared the outcomes of living donor transplant and surgical resection using propensity score method. Although there was no survival benefit between either treatment options, LTx provided significantly reduced recurrence rate than surgical resection (9% *versus* 21%).

Tumour ablation is an alternative to surgical resection for early stage HCC patients who are not suitable for surgery. It can be achieved by application of chemical agents (alcohol or acetic acid) or by change in temperature (radiofrequency, microwave, laser, and cryoablation).

Percutaneous Ethanol Injection (PEI)

PEI is suggested for the treatment of nodular HCC ≤ 5cm in diameter, and can achieve necrosis of 90%-100% in HCC ≤ 2cm, 70% in 2cm-3cm and up to 50% in HCC of 3cm-5cm [24]. PEI requires repeated injection on separate days and is not effective in HCC patients with tumours larger than 3cm because the injected ethanol cannot penetrate the entire tumour volume. There is no statistically significant difference in the 5-year survival and recurrence rates compared to surgical resection in patients with tumour size < 3cm [24, 25]. However, Huang GT *et al.* [25] reported better survival after surgery in patients with HCC tumours > 3cm. A major limitation of PEI is the high rate of recurrence (33%-43%) [26].

Percutaneous Acetic Acid Injection (PAI)

PAI is more effective than PEI as acetic acid has a better diffusion capacity. It is also cheap and widely available. A smaller volume of acetic acid achieves the same level of ablation as ethanol and with fewer treatment sessions. It is ideally performed on HCC smaller than 3cm in size. The local tumour recurrence rates for 1 year and 3 years are 51% and 74% respectively. The survival rate at 1 and 3 years is 84% and 51%, respectively [27]. Some studies report a lower local recurrence rate for PAI (8%) compared to PEI (37%). No statistically significant difference have been reported in survival outcomes between PAI and PEI [28].

Radiofrequency Ablation (RFA)

RFA is the most commonly used ablation technique worldwide, replacing PEI as the therapy of choice for early HCC (< 3cm). It induces thermal injury to the hepatic tissue through electromagnetic energy. Compared to PEI, it requires fewer treatment sessions to achieve comparable anti-tumoural effects. Several randomised control trials have also reported a lower recurrence rate compared to PIE (2 year local recurrence rate: 2%-18% *versus* 11%-45%, respectively) [29, 30]. The highest 5-year survival rate (51%-64%) has been observed in Child-Pugh A patients with early-stage HCC. Several studies have reported comparable OS rates between RFA and surgical resection [31, 32] but with surgical resection having better disease-free survival [33]. Higher costs and complications involving pleural effusion and peritoneal bleeding are the major drawbacks of RFA [24].

Microwave Ablation (MWA)

MWA involves the use of microwave energy that causes vibration of water molecules in tissues producing heat resulting in cell death. It was previously used during liver surgery to control bleeding from ruptured HCC and for liver resection. MWA can achieve high tissue temperatures leading to enhanced efficacy of ablation compared to RFA. Additionally, MWA is not affected by 'heat-sink' effects next to major blood vessels, unlike RFA, and can ablate tumours next to major blood vessels [34]. Due to its enhanced efficacy and shorter time to achieve ablations, MWA has been used to treat both primary and metastatic HCC tumours. Ding J *et al.* [35] compared RFA and MWA in 198 HCC patients and found similar disease-free survival and cumulative survival rates between the two groups. Zhang L *et al.* [36] also found that RFA and MWA had equivalent OS and recurrence rates.

Percutaneous Laser Ablation (PLA)

PLA uses laser light to induce tissue hyperthermia in tumours. It is a highly effective treatment in HCC with a tumour size of ≤4cm or smaller. Two variables, tumour size and tumour location, not only affect the extent of complete tumour ablation but also the number of treatment sessions required to obtain tumour necrosis [37]. Pacell C *et al.* [37] has reported about 90% tumour ablation with efficacy decreasing with increase in tumour size (> 3cm) [37]. Ferrari FS *et al.* [38] compared PLA and RFA in a prospective randomized study of 81 cirrhotic patients with HCC. Although RFA had improved OS as compared to PLA at 1, 3 and 5 years (92.2% *versus* 88.6%, 75.0% *versus* 70.4%, 40.9% *versus* 22.9%; respectively), the difference was not statistically significant.

Cryoablation

Cryoablation therapy takes advantage of the extreme cold temperature of liquid nitrogen or argon gas to kill cancer tissue. It can achieve complete ablation rates of 81.2%, 99.4%, 94.4%, and 45.6% in all tumours, tumours < 3cm, tumours < 5cm, and tumours > 5cm, respectively [39, 40]. In comparison to RFA and MWA, cryoablation has shown to provide improved local control for HCC > 2cm [41]. In a multicentre randomised control trial (registered as Chinese domestic clinical trial, 20071203T) in China involving HCC patients with tumours < 4cm, Wanc C *et al.* [42] reported cryoablation to be as effective and have similar 5-year OS rate as RFA.

Trans-Arterial Therapies and Systemic Chemotherapy

The liver has a dual blood supply from the hepatic artery and the portal vein. HCC receives a majority of blood supply from the hepatic artery resulting in neo-angiogenesis. Trans-arterial therapy takes advantage of the vast blood supply to the HCC by administration of cytotoxic drugs/embolizing agents to the tumour without affecting hepatic blood supply. Trans-arterial therapies include TACE, trans-arterial chemotherapy (TAC), and trans-arterial radioembolization (TART).

TACE

TACE is the standard treatment option for HCC patients with compensated liver function and large single nodule or multifocal HCC (< 5cm). The main factors that preclude TACE include extra-hepatic spread, portal vein thrombosis, and decompensated liver cirrhosis [43]. It is a twin procedure involving delivery of high doses of chemotherapeutic drugs followed by embolization to allow prolonged retention of the drugs in the tumour leading to ischemic necrosis and death. Survival outcomes of TACE have been studied extensively. In 2002, a randomised controlled trial in Hong Kong looked into the survival benefit of TACE in unresectable HCC showing significantly enhanced actuarial survival (1 year, 57%; 2 years, 31%; 3 years, 26%) than in the control group which received symptomatic treatment (1 year, 32%; 2 years, 11%; 3 years, 3%) [44]. However, Doffoël M *et al.* [45] did not report improved survival benefit of TACE. Despite this, in the largest cohort study involving 8,510 HCC patients with unresectable HCC, Takayasu K *et al.* [46] showed a median survival of 34 months with a survival benefit at 1, 3, 5 and 7 year as 82%, 47%, 26% and 16%, respectively. A study from India in which TACE was conducted on HCC with large tumour size (median size 6.3cm $\pm$ 3.92cm) depicted cumulative survival rate at 1, 2, 3 years as 66%,47% and 36.4% respectively [47]. TACE has become an established therapeutic option for intermediate stage of HCC. In the future additional studies need to investigate the impact on survival resulting from different type or combination of chemotherapeutic agents, as well as the embolizing medium.

TAC

TAC is used for the treatment of HCC patients with portal vein thrombosis and involves only the injection of chemotherapeutic drugs with no subsequent embolization. No difference in survival has been reported between TACE and TAC [48]. A meta-analysis by Leung DA *et al.* [49], suggested lack of clinical benefit from TAC. Thus, TAC is not the preferred choice of treatment.

TART

TART refers to the percutaneous intra-arterial injection of radiation without causing ischemia. β-Radiation from radioactive yttrium-loaded glass or resin particles is applied through arteries that feed the tumour. Two retrospective studies depicted similar effectiveness and toxicity for TART and TACE [50, 51]. In a recent retrospective study, Ozkan G *et al.* [52] reported TART to have the same survival benefit as TACE in advanced HCC patients who cannot undergo TACE due to portal vein thrombosis. However, TART is expensive and this may limit its application.

Systematic Chemotherapy

Systemic chemotherapeutic agents including cisplatin, doxorubicin (DOX), 5-fluoroucil (5-FU), gemcitabine or combined regimens for palliative care are not recommended for HCC patients with advanced tumours because they are associated with low response rates (0-18%) with no clear impact on survival. Furthermore, underlying cirrhosis enhances the toxicity of chemotherapeutic drugs [53, 54]. The reasons for chemoresistance are poorly understood but likely reasons include overexpression of multidrug-resistance protein (high ATP-binding cassette (ABC) [55], and loss of expression of tumour suppressor genes (p53, PTEN) [56].

In a phase III randomised control trial (ClinicalTrials.gov number, NCT00012324), a recent cytotoxic agent, nolatrexed, showed an inferior median OS compared with DOX (22.3 weeks *versus* 32.3 weeks, $P=0.0068$). Side effects including grade 3 and 4 stomatitis, vomiting, diarrhoea, and thrombocytopenia were more common in patients treated with nolatrexed and consequently more patients were withdrawn from nolatrexed due to toxicity than due to doxorubicin [57].

A large randomised control trial that compared combination therapy of cisplatin, interferonα2b/DOX/5-FU (PIAF) *versus* DOX alone did not show any statistically significant difference in OS (8.67 months *versus* 6.83 months, $P=0.83$). However, PIAF was associated with a significantly higher rate of myelotoxixity compared to DOX alone [54]. Similarly, in another randomised control study (NCT00471965) conducted in Asia, no statistically significant difference in OS was reported between oxaliplatin plus 5-FU/leucovorin (FOLFOX4) *versus* DOX (6.40 months *versus* 4.97 months, $P=0.07$) [58]. Therefore, in the absence of any survival benefit along with treatment-related toxicity, single or combined regimens are not recommended for treatment of advanced HCC.

Targeted Therapies

HCC is characterized by multiple epigenetic and genetic changes that result in uncontrolled growth of hepatocytes. Several signalling pathways, oncogenes, growth factors and their receptors are being considered and are going through clinical trials for their potential therapeutic effect for systemic targeted therapies. Table **2** lists completed phase III clinical trials of some systemic targeted agents in HCC.

Table 2. Completed phase III clinical trials of some systemic targeted agents in HCC.

Comparison	Clinical Name and Study Number	Patients, *n*	OS	*P* Value	Ref
Nolatrexed *versus* doxorubicin	--, NCT00012324	222 *versus* 222	22.3 weeks *versus* 32.3 weeks	*P*=0.0068	[57]
Sorafenib *versus* placebo	SHARP trial, NCT00105443	299 *versus* 303	10.7 months *versus* 7.9 months	*P*<0.001	[59]
Sorafenib *versus* placebo	Asia Pacific trial, NCT00492752	150 *versus* 76	6.5 months *versus* 4.2 months	*P*<0.014	[60]
Sunitinib *versus* sorafenib	--, NCT00699374	530 *versus* 544	7.9 months *versus* 10.2 months	*P*=0.0014	[61]
Brivanib *versus* sorafenib	BRISK-PS trial, NCT01108705	263 *versus* 132	9.4 months *versus* 8.2 months	*P*=0.33	[62]
Brivanib *versus* sorafenib	BRISK-FL trial, NCT00858871	577 *versus* 578	9.5 months *versus* 9.9 months	*P*=0.31	[63]
Linifanib *versus* sorafenib	LIGHT trial, NCT01009593	517 *versus* 518	9.1 months *versus* 9.8 months	*P*<0.001	[64]
Everolimus *versus* placebo	EVOLVE-1 trial, NCT01035229	362 *versus* 184	7.6 months *versus* 7.3 months	*P*=0.68	[65]

--: no name assigned; OS: overall survival; NCT: ClinicalTrials.gov number.

Anti-angiogenic Pathway

With HCC being a highly vascular tumour, it is important to target angiogenic growth factors such as vascular endothelial growth factor receptor (VEGFR), fibroblast growth factor receptor (FGFR), and platelet-derived growth factor receptor (PDGFR), whose increased expression have been associated to poor survival [66]. Fig. (**2**) demonstrates some of the signalling pathways and receptors targeted for treatment of HCC.

Sorafenib

Sorafenib is an orally administered multi-kinase inhibitor with anti-angiogenic and anti-proliferative activities, though its exact mechanism remains unknown. Currently, sorafenib is the only drug approved for treatment of advanced HCC as well as those intolerant to TACE. This is based on results from two phase III randomised placebo-controlled trials, the SHARP trial (NCT00105443) [59] and the Asia Pacific trial (NCT00492752) [60]. In the SHARP trial, sorafenib significantly increased the OS of advanced HCC patients from 7.9 months to 10.7 months (*P*<0.001) and the time to progression (TTP) from 2.8 months to 5.5 months (*P*<0.001). The Asia Pacific trial reported similar results with and OS and TTP being enhanced from 4.2 months to 6.5 months (*P*<0.014) and from 1.4

months to 2.8 months (P=0.0005), respectively. The reason for the reduced OS in the Asia Pacific trial could possibly be due to differences in HCC patient aetiology. In the SHARP trail, 12% of patients had baseline HBV compared to 73.0% in the Asia Pacific trial. Additionally, 8.4% of HCC patients in the Asia Pacific trial had baseline HCV infection compared to 30% in the SHARP trial.

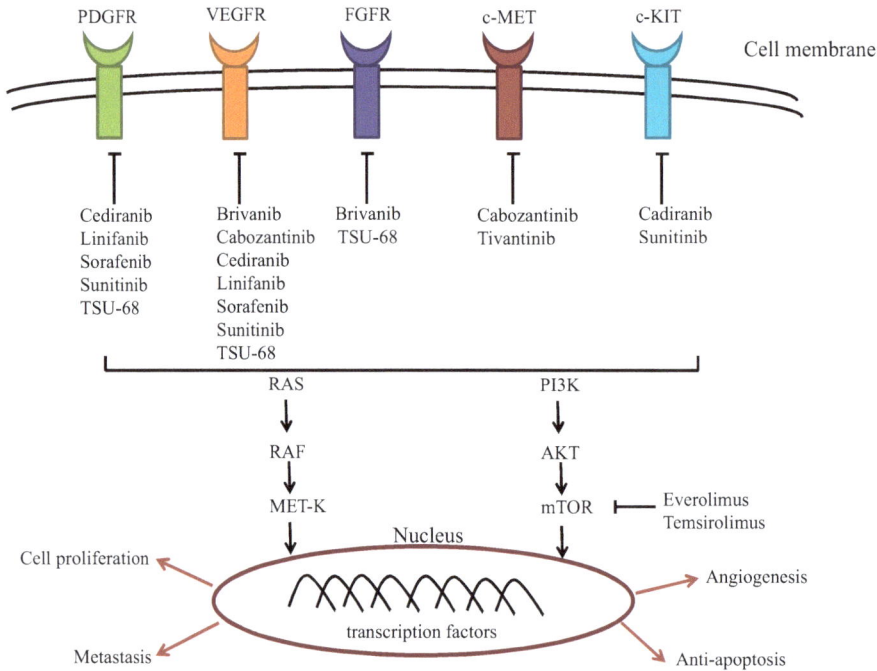

Fig. (2). Signalling pathways and molecular targets of various targeted therapies under investigation for treatment of HCC. PDGFR: platelet-derived growth factor receptor; VEGFR: vascular endothelial growth factor receptor; FGFR: fibroblast growth factor receptor.

Sorafenib is currently being studied as an adjuvant after resection, and in combination with TACE for intermediate HCC. In a recently completed phase III placebo-controlled, double-blind trial (STORM, NCT00692770), the effect of sorafenib as an adjuvant treatment after surgery/ablation to prevent HCC recurrence was investigated [67]. The results of this study have not been published yet but they will provide important findings on the efficacy of sorafenib to prevent HCC recurrence in early stage HCC.

Controversial results have been observed in studies evaluating the effects of sorafenib with TACE. Two phase II trials have reported promising efficacy of

TACE and sorafenib in patients with unresectable HCC [68, 69]. In a small prospective, single-centre, placebo-controlled, randomized, double-blind clinical study, Sansonno D *et al.* [70] demonstrated significantly longer TTP in patients with intermediate stage HCC who underwent conventional TACE procedure followed by sorafenib treatment compared to patients who only received TACE plus placebo (9.2 months *versus* 4.9 month, $P < .001$). The small sample size (31 *versus* 31) limits the evidence level and the results of this study need to be confirmed in a larger phase III clinical trial with follow-up period long enough to evaluate an OS advantage. However, in a randomised phase III trial (NCT00494299) of sorafenib after TACE, sorafenib did not significantly enhance TTP compared to placebo (5.4 months *versus* 3.7 months, $P=0.252$) [71]. The researchers attributed the poor response to sorafenib to either prolonged delay in administration of sorafenib after TACE (a lag time of > 9 weeks) and/or low sorafenib dose. Subsequently another trial (TACTICS, NCT01217034) is underway with a different lag time (3 days -21 days). In a propensity score matching study involving patients with advanced HCC, Hu H *et al.* [72] observed significantly better OS and TTP for patients undergoing TACE with sorafenib *versus* TACE monotherapy. The median OS and TTP were 7.0 months *versus* 4.9 months ($P=0.003$), and 2.6 months *versus* 1.9 months ($P=0.001$), respectively. This study showed that combination therapy of sorafenib with TACE was well tolerated and effective than TACE alone. Overall further randomized control trials are needed to evaluate the effectiveness, the timing of sorafenib administration after TACE, and identify which patients will benefit from the combination therapy of TACE and sorafenib.

Sunitinib

Sunitinib is an oral multi-targeted receptor kinase inhibitor with activity against VEGFR, PDGFR, c-KIT and various other kinases, though its mechanism of action remains unknown. It has been approved for the treatment of renal cell carcinoma (RCC), and imatinib-resistant gastrointestinal stromal tumours (GIST). In two phase II studies of sunitinib in patients with advanced HCC, patients received 50mg daily of sunitinib orally, 4 weeks on and two weeks off. However, both studies reported high toxicity, with one study reporting treatment-related deaths in 10% of patients (4, n=37) and another study reporting grade 3/4 adverse effects in 80% of patients [73, 74]. The high toxicity of sunitinib may be a result of the many different receptors it targets. A phase II study involving continuous sunitinib treatment (37.5mg daily) demonstrated progression-free survival at 12 weeks of 33.3% [75]. However, a multicentre phase III trial (NCT00699374) compared sunitinib to sorafenib as the first-line of treatment for advanced HCC. Patients were administered 37.5mg of sunitinib once daily or 400mg of sorafenib twice a day. This trial ended prematurely due to higher incidence of adverse side effects in the sunitinib arm. Furthermore, sunitinib did not give a superior advantage over sorafenib in terms of OS (7.9 months *versus* 10.2 months, P=0.0014) [61]. Consequently, as a result of its high incidence of toxicity and inferior outcomes of patients, sunitinib is not considered as a therapeutic option for HCC.

Brivanib

Brivanib is a dual VEGFR and FGFR inhibitor. Preclinical studies have shown that brivanib has potent anti-tumour activity suppressing patient-derived xenograft HCC models resistant to sorafenib [76]. However, several phase III studies for the treatment of HCC with brivanib have yielded negative results. A multicentre, double-blind, randomized, placebo-controlled trial (BRISK-PS, NCT01108705) assessed brivanib in advanced HCC patients who were intolerant to sorafenib or for whom sorafenib had failed [62]. The median OS was 9.4 months for those given brivanib and 8.2 months for those given placebo (P=0.33). However, there was difference in the median TTP (4.2 months for patients with brivanib *versus* 2.7 months for patients given placebo). Thus, patients who had been treated with sorafenib did not show improved OS after brivanib treatment. Another randomized, double-blind, phase III trial (BRISK-FL, NCT00858871) compared brivanib with sorafenib as first-line treatment for advanced HCC. This study did not meet its primary end point of OS noninferiority for brivanib *versus* sorafenib, yielding a median OS of 9.9 months for patients with sorafenib and 9.5 months for patients with brivanib (P=0.31) [63]. TTP were similar in both arms. Both these studies did not improve the OS for patients with advanced HCC. Recently Kudo M *et al.* [77] reported that brivanib as an adjuvant to TACE did not improve OS (26.4 months for brivanib and TACE *versus* 26.1 months for TACE, P=0.53).

Linifanib

Linifanib is a multi-targeted tyrosine kinase inhibitor inhibiting VEGFR and PDGFR families. In a recently concluded open-label phase III trial (LIGHT trial, NCT01009593) evaluating efficacy and tolerability of linifanib *versus* sorafenib in advanced HCC, Caiban C *et al.* [64] reported similar OS for the two (9.1 months for linifanib and 9.8 months for sorafinib, P<0.001). Patients were administered either linifanib 17.5 mg once daily or sorafenib 400 mg twice daily.

Other Kinase Inhibitors

TSU-68 inhibits VEGFR, FGFR and PDGFR and has demonstrated promising preliminary efficacy in a phase I/II trial (NCT00784290) of advanced HCC yielding TTP of 2.1 months, and median OS of 13.1 months [78]. Another trial (JapicCTI-101087, registered with Japanese Pharmaceutical Information Centre) combining TSU-68 with TACE in advanced HCC patients reported a trend towards prolonged progression free survival (PFS) with TSU-68 treatment after a single session of TACE but this was not statistically significant [79].

Cediranib is another multi-targeted tyrosine kinase inhibitor of VEGFR, PDGFR, c-KIT. In a phase II clinical trial (NCT00238394), at 45 mg per day cediranib was toxic and yielded OS of 5.8 months and TTP of 2.8 months [80]. In a subsequent phase II study (NCT00427973) using a smaller dosage (30 mg per day), cediranib showed antitumor efficacy in advanced HCC with a favourable OS of 11.7 months compared to 5.8 months at 45 mg per day [81]. The difference in OS at the two cediranib dosages may be a result of longer duration of treatment with 30 mg per day and bias in patient selection may have also been a factor.

c-Met Inhibitors

Stimulation of hepatocyte growth factor (HGF)/c-MET signalling pathway plays an important role in the development of various solid cancers, including HCC, through activation of a cascade reaction of Ras/Raf/Mek/ERk and PI3K/AKT resulting in tumour growth, invasion and resistance to apoptosis. In HCC, activation of HGF/c-MET pathway has been associated to poor prognosis [82].

Tivantinib is a selective non-ATP competitive inhibitor of c-MET. Its use as a second-line treatment for advanced HCC has been evaluated in a multicentre, randomised, placebo-controlled, double-blind, phase II study (NCT00988741) [83]. Patients were initially given 360 mg twice-daily but this was reduced to 240 mg daily because of high incidence of neutropenia. The study showed a modest improvement in TTP from 1.4 months to 1.6 months (P=0.04), favouring the tivantinib group. Furthermore important results from this trial were obtained from sub-group analysis of c-MET expression. HCC tumours expressing high levels of c-MET (high expression was regarded as ≥2+ in ≥50% of tumour cells by immunohistochemical analysis), had improved OS (7.2 months *versus* 3.8 months, P=0.01) and longer median TTP (2.7 months *versus* 1.4 months, P=0.03) when administered tivantinib than when given a placebo. c-MET status may serve as a potential predictive marker to select patients most likely to benefit from treatment. A large, randomized, double-blind, confirmatory phase III trial (METIV-HCC, NCT 01755767) is underway to assess the effect of tivantinib on OS in HCC patients with c-MET expression.

Cabozantinib is an oral multi-targeted tyrosine kinase inhibitor with activity against c-MET, and VEGFR. *In vitro* and *in vivo* data in HCC cell lines and mouse xenograft model indicated that high levels of phosphorylated MET (p-MET) are associated with resistance to adjuvant sorafenib treatment and that cabozantinib had significant anti-tumour activity [84]. Cabozantinib blocked HGF stimulated MET pathway and inhibited migration and invasion of HCC cells. Furthermore, cabozantinib reduced metastatic lesions in the lung and liver in an experimental metastatic mouse model. These results also show potential of c-MET expression as a biomarker for predicting response to cabozantinib in adjuvant sorafenib resistant tumours. Patients are currently being recruited for a phase III, randomized, double-blind, controlled study of cabozantinib *versus* placebo in HCC patients who have received prior sorafenib (NCT01908426).

mTOR Inhibitors

mTOR signalling is upregulated in 40%-45% of HCC and is associated to bad prognosis, poorly differentiated tumours, and earlier recurrence [85, 86]. Preclinical studies have reported effective inhibition of cell proliferation, tumour growth and metastasis in HCC tumour models by mTOR inhibitors [87]. Currently available mTOR inhibitors, everolimus and temsirolimus, were initially developed for immunosuppressive treatment after liver transplantation rather than cancer treatment.

Everolimus is an oral mTOR inhibitor. Preclinical studies have demonstrated that everolimus inhibits tumour growth in xenograft models of advanced HCC [87]. Toxicity and efficacy of everolimus was tested in 28 advanced HCC patients in a phase I/II study (NCT00516165). Daily dosage of 5 mg or 10 mg per day was well tolerated in Phase I, yielding a medium PFS and OS of 3.8 months and 8.4 months respectively. In phase II, 25 HCC patients, most of whom had prior systemic therapy, were given 10 mg per day but this part of the study could not proceed to completion as only two patients were progression free for 24 weeks [88]. Although everolimus was well tolerated and preliminary antitumor activity was observed with everolimus in patients with advanced HCC, important limitations of the study included small sample size and lack of a randomized control. In a phase III, randomized, double-blind study (EVOLVE-1, NCT01035229), Zhu Ax *et al.* [65] assessed the efficacy of everolimus in patients with advanced HCC for whom sorafenib treatment had failed. Results indicated that everolimus failed to improve OS (7.6 months with everolimus, 7.3 months with placebo, $P=0.68$) [65]. However, a recent study suggested the loss of tuberous sclerosis complex 2 (TSC2) as a predictive biomarker for response to everolimus. Analysis of TSC2 status in HCC samples collected in the EVOLVE-1 clinical trial (NCT01035229) by immunohistochemical analysis, Huynh H *et al.* [89] identified 10.8% (15/139) of samples to have low or undetectable levels of TSC2 and longer OS than compared to placebo. A larger study is required to validate the potential of TSC2 to predict response to everolimus.

Similarly, temsirolimus, an intravenously administered mTOR inhibitor, did not yield encouraging results when used in monotherapy or in combination with sorafenib or bevacizumab. mTOR inhibitors are immunosuppressive agents and a recently concluded phase III trial (NCT00355862) looked into the effect of mTOR inhibitor (sirolimus) for patients with advanced HCC, after liver transplantation. The results of this study are yet to be published [90].

Immune Based and Antiviral Therapies

Immune Based Therapy

The job of the immune system is to recognize and destroy tumour cells. However cancer cells are able to avoid detection and destruction by the immune system. Immunotherapy attempts to boost the body's immune response to target tumour cells. One of the promising approaches to activate antitumor activity is the blockade of immune checkpoints which are a network of inhibitory pathways that are important in maintaining the amplitude and duration of immune response of T cells. Under normal physiological conditions, immune checkpoints are critical for maintenance of self-tolerance and protection of tissues from damage during pathogenic infection. Recent data suggests that tumours take-over some immune checkpoints as a way to develop immune resistance. Manipulation of the inhibitory checkpoints by way of monoclonal antibodies or soluble receptors offer potential therapeutic strategies for enhancing T cell activity against tumour growth [91].

Monoclonal antibody directed against CTLA4, ipilimumab, is the first checkpoint-blocking antibody to be approved by the Food and Drug Administration (FDA) for treatment of advanced melanoma after it demonstrated improved survival benefit [92]. In a small pilot clinical trial with 21 patients with metastatic HCV-related HCC (HCV-HCC), tremelimumab (CTLA4 monoclonal antibody), induced a significant decrease in viral load and showed promising partial response rate and disease control rate of 17.6% and 76.4%, respectively. Programed death-1 (PD-1) is another immune checkpoint receptor that inhibits T-cell activation upon binding to PD ligands (PDL)-1 and PDL-2. PDL-1 is overexpressed in HCC and preclinical data has suggested PD-1 and PDL-1 to suppress HCC growth *in vivo* [93], suggesting a potential therapeutic target. Clinical trials on PD-1 (nivolumab, NCT01658878) and PDL-1 (MED14736, NCT01693562) blockers are underway in advanced HCC patients. In addition these agents will also be investigated as antivirals and for early stages of HCC within the context of ablation and TACE.

Antiviral Therapy

Evidence from several studies has shown that high serum levels of HBV DNA ($\geq$10,000 copies/mL) are associated with cirrhosis and HBV related HCC (HBV-HCC) [94 - 97]. Integration of HBV gene into the host genome results in changes in host genome gene expression contributing to the development of carcinogenesis. Furthermore, the viral protein HBx is critical for hepato-carcinogenesis as it affects several signalling pathways and genes involved in proliferation, inflammation, immune response, and oncogenesis. Since the presence and replication of HBV is crucial for of HBV-HCC, suppression of viral replication is a reasonable target for the prevention of HCC. Sustained HBV suppression has been shown to be associated with long-term survival [98]. However, HBV reactivation is common after curative resection for HBV-HCC and might influence prognosis [99]. Postoperative antiviral treatment offers potential to reduce viral load and improve postoperative prognosis.

Currently approved treatment for viral infection in HBV-HCC include interferon-α (IFN-α) and nucleotide analogues (NA), including lamivudine, entecavir, telbivudine, and adefovir-dipivoxil.

IFN-α

In a prospective study analysing IFN-α therapy in patients with HBV positive cirrhosis and HCC who underwent ablation, Someya T *et al.* [100] reported a decrease in tumour recurrence in patients with HBV-related cirrhosis. Furthermore, a randomised controlled trial (NCT00234182) investigated the prognostic effect of interferon therapy following hepatic resection. Forty patients with HBV-HCC after curative hepatic resection were treated with IFN-α three times weekly for 16 weeks compared to non-treated control group. The IFN group yielded 1 and 5 year survival rates of 97% and 79%, respectively compared to 85% and 60% in the control group (P=0.137). In a subset analysis, interferon therapy had no effect on 5 year survival benefit for early stage HCC (pTNM I or II, P=0.087) but prevented recurrence and improved survival in late stage HCC (pTNM, III/IVA, P=0.038) [101]. Similarly in a larger randomised clinical trial involving HBV-HCC patients, Sun HC *et al.* [102] also reported improved OS compared to the control group (63.8 months *versus* 38.8 months, P=0.0003). However, contrary to these results a recent phase III randomised study (NCT00149565) of IFN-α2b conducted in Taiwan did not demonstrate improved postoperative recurrence in HBV-HCC and HCV-HCC following curative resection [103]. These studies suggest an unclear role of IFN-α in HCC and further studies are warranted.

NA

NA inhibits HBV replication, but there is conflicting data on their potential to reduce the incidence of HBV-HCC. Lamivudine is a first generation NA widely used to treat patients with hepatitis B. There has only been one randomized controlled clinical trial involving chronic hepatitis patients where lamivudine was found to significantly reduce the risk of HCC compared to placebo (3.9% *versus* 7.4%, *P*=0.047) [104]. The effect of lamivudine on overall survival and HCC recurrence has also been investigated in several clinical trials. Some studies failed to demonstrate any beneficial impact of adjuvant NA [105 - 107] while others reported significant improvement on recurrence-free survival and OS [108 - 110]. In a randomised clinical trial (registered with Chinese Clinical Trial Registry, ChiCTR-TRC-08000172), antiviral therapy yielded a better 2-year overall (94% *versus* 62%) and recurrence-free (56% *versus* 20%) survival compared with no NA therapy [108]. Telbivudine and entecavir have shown greater potency than lamivudine against HBV. In a double-blind phase III trial (NCT00057265), telbivudine demonstrated greater viral suppression and resistance compared to lamivudine [111]. Likewise, in phase II (NCT00035633) and subsequent phase III clinical trials, entecavir showed a significantly higher rate of histologic, virologic, and biochemical improvement compared to lamivudine [112, 113]. Combination therapy of NAs has thus far not demonstrated additive viral suppression. Combination of lamivudine and adefovir-dipivoxil *versus* lamivudine alone in chronic hepatitis B (CHB) patients yielded similar virological suppression in both treatment arms. However, lamivudine resistance rate at two years was lower in the combination group compared to the group that received lamivudine alone [114]. Lai CL *et al.* [115] studied lamivudine and telbivudine both as monotherapy as well as combination therapy in CHB patients. Drug resistance was observed in 5% of patients in the telbivudine group compared to 12% rate of resistance in the combination group of lamivudine and telbivudine.

Approval of potent NAs, such as telbivudine and entecavir has been a milestone in CHB treatment but the long-term use of NAs has been hindered by the development of drug-resistant mutants [116].

For HCV-HCC, successful treatment results in sustained virologic response (SVR), which is the absence of viral RNA in blood 24 weeks after completion of therapy. SVR is associated with reduced rate of HCC and liver decompensation, and improved survival. The current standard treatment includes 24-48 weeks of pegylated IFNα (pegINFα) in combination with ribavirin (RBV). Both of these drugs act on multiple nonspecific pathways that affect immune response. HCV-HCC patients with genotype 1 and 2 have achieved the highest SVR of 80% after 24 weeks of therapy. However, HCV-HCC patients with genotype 1 are the most difficult to treat because their SVR is only 40% following 48 weeks of therapy. Both these drugs have severe side effects and many patients treated with them discontinue the therapy. For these reasons, new therapies called direct-acting antiviral agents (DAA) are focusing on targeting the HCV viral life cycle for direct inhibition of viral production [117].

Unlike the HBV, HCV cannot integrate into the host genome. The various stages of the HCV life cycle offer several potential therapeutic targets. At the first step of the life cycle, the virus attaches to the hepatocyte cell surface where the virus and the cell membrane fuse to allow entry of virus *via* endocytosis. Upon release of the nucleocapsid into the cytoplasm, positive-strand RNA is released into the cytoplasm where it is translated into polyprotein. The polyprotein undergoes proteolytical processing by viral and cellular proteases, followed by viral replication, assembly and release [118, 119].

Viral Entry

Several monoclonal and polyclonal antibodies are being investigated to prevent attachment of viral particles to the cell receptor or to prevent viral entry. HCV AB68, HCV Ab6865 and bavituximab are in clinical trials [120].

Translation

The internal ribosome entry site (IRES), located on the 5'UTR region of the virus, and regulates HCV translation. The efficiency of the translation is affected by NS4A and NS5A proteins. Early-phase studies are underway to block this step using antisense oligonucleotides [121].

Post-Translational Processing

Following translation of the viral genome the proteins undergo post-translational processing mainly by NS2-2 protease and NS3/4A protease. The 2 most studied NS3/4A inhibitors for DAA therapy include boceprevir and telaprevir [122].

Boceprevir

In a phase II randomised multicentre study (SPRINT-1, NCT00423670) of treatment-naïve HCV-HCC patients, 2 treatment groups received boceprevir in combination with pegIFNα-2b and RBV for 28 weeks (group 1) or 48 weeks (group 2). The control group received pegIFNα-2b and RBV for 48 weeks. Treatment groups 1 and 2 achieved SVR of 54% and 67% respectively compared to SVR rate of 38% in the control group [123].

In another phase III study, RESPOND-2 (NCT00708500), boceprevir was assessed in patients who had relapsed or were not responsive to standard treatment. Group 1 included a control group (pegIFNα-2b and RBV for 48 weeks). Group 2 received pegIFNα-2b and RBV for 4 weeks followed by response guided therapy with 800mg boceprebir plus pegIFNα-2b and RBV for 33 weeks. Group 3 received 4 weeks of pegIFNα-2b and RBV followed by 44 weeks of boceprebir plus pegIFNα-2b and RBV. The SVR in patients with prior relapse were 29% in group 1, 69% in group 2 and 75% in group 3. Among patients with prior nonresponse, the corresponding SVR rates were 7% *versus* 40% and 52%, respectively. Thus, results favouring the use of boceprevir in difficult-to-treat patients [124].

Telaprevir

Several phase III studies have assessed the significance of telaprevir over standard treatment.

In the ADVANCE trial (NCT00627926), telaprevir with pegIFNα-2b and RBV, as compared with pegIFNα-2b and RBV alone, was associated with significantly improved rates of SVR (79% and 44% respectively) in patients who had not received previous treatment [125].

Like the boceprevir RESPOND trial, in the REALIZE trial (NCT00703118) telaprevir also demonstrated improved SVR rates in patients who were not responsive to pegIFNα-2b and RBV alone or those who had relapsed. In patients with relapse, addition of telaprevir to pegIFNα-2b and RBV achieved SVR rates of 83% compared to 24% in the control group (pegIFNα-2b and RBV only). Similarly, patients who were not responsive to pegIFNα-2b and RBV alone achieved SVR of 41% following addition of telaprevir compared to 9% in the control group [126].

Although boceprevir and telaprevir offer improved SVR rates in combination with pegIFNα-2b and RBV, their use is restricted due to treatment-related adverse side-effects such as anaemia and severe rash. Several mutations conferring resistance to boceprevir and telaprevir have also been reported in the blood of HCV-infected patients [127, 128]. Whether these mutations will affect successful re-treatment with these drugs has not been clearly investigated.

Replication

After translation of the viral genome, viral replication is mediated by NS5B polymerase, which is another important target of therapy. NS5B polymerase inhibitors fall into two categories, the nucleos(t)ide inhibitors and the non-nucleos(t)ide inhibitors.

Recently sofosbuvir, a nucleotide inhibitor, was approved as a highly potent inhibitor of NS5B polymerase. Sofosbuvir is taken orally and offers a high barrier to resistance [129]. Its efficacy has been reported in several phase III clinical trials. In the NEUTRINO (NCT01641640) study, sofosbuvir in combination with pegIFNα-2b and RBV for 12 weeks in treatment naïve patients, resulted in 90% SVR rate, which was statistically superior to control SVR rate of 60% [130]. In another phase III study (FUSION, NCT01604850), patients who were not responsive to pegIFNα-2b or for whom treatment with pegIFNα-2b was not an option, sofosbuvir in combination with RBV yielded a higher SVR rate of 78%, as compared with 0% with placebo [131].

BMS-791325 is a non-nucleoside inhibitor that has shown to achieve a sustained SVR in early-phase studies [132]. This drug is in clinical trials in combination with other DAAs.

Although DAAs offer an opportunity to reduce HCC, recent reports suggest of a high rate of HCC recurrence in patients on antiviral therapies. A large-scale investigation is warranted to assess this risk [133, 134]. Fig. (**3**) summarizes the different kinds of non-surgical therapies that have been investigated in HCC.

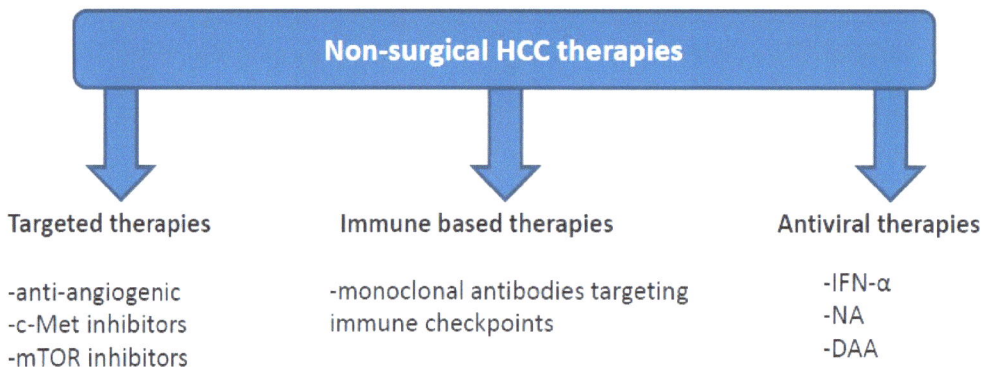

Fig. (3). A summary of the different HCC therapies available or under investigation. IFN-α: interferon-α; NA: nucleotide analogues; DAA: direct-acting antiviral agents.

CONCLUDING REMARKS

HCC is a complex disease with a pathogenesis including HBV and HCV infections as well as underlying cirrhosis. Thus effective treatment of HCC would require simultaneous treatment of hepatitis, cirrhosis and cancer. Currently for early HCC patients, the only curative therapies include hepatic resection or liver transplantation. Unfortunately, a large majority of HCC patients are not suitable for these therapies and palliative treatment is the only option. For patients with intermediate HCC, surgical resection offers the only potential for cure. Other options include TACE or RFA.

For advanced HCC, sorafenib remains the only standard therapy for advanced HCC even though it only provides a modest survival benefit. Nevertheless, its development highlights the importance of molecular targeted therapies in the treatment of chemo-resistant HCC. At present numerous agents targeting angiogenesis, immune response *etc.* show promising results in preclinical studies and some of the agents are under phase III development. However, in the absence of biomarkers that can predict response to molecularly targeted, phase III clinical trials risk disappointing results if wrong patients are selected. In addition, several signalling pathways are activated in HCC and no single dominant pathway has been identified in hepatocarcinogenesis. Further studies are also warranted to evaluate the use of neoadjuvant/adjuvant therapies to decrease recurrence following resection or ablation, combinations of systemic therapies, and combinations of systemic targeted therapies. In the era of molecular targeted therapies, rational approach based on cost, toxicity, quality of life and survival is needed to guide both patients and physicians. To conclude, treatment of HCC patients remains a major challenge and requires a multidisciplinary approach.

CONFLICT OF INTEREST

The authors declares no conflict of interest, financial or otherwise.

ACKNOWLEDGEMENTS

Declared none.

REFERENCES

[1]   Torre LA, Bray F, Siegel RL, Ferlay J, Lortet-Tieulent J, Jemal A. Global cancer statistics, 2012. CA Cancer J Clin 2015; 65(2): 87-108.
[http://dx.doi.org/10.3322/caac.21262] [PMID: 25651787]

[2]   Altekruse SF, McGlynn KA, Reichman ME. Hepatocellular carcinoma incidence, mortality, and survival trends in the United States from 1975 to 2005. J Clin Oncol 2009; 27(9): 1485-91.
[http://dx.doi.org/10.1200/JCO.2008.20.7753] [PMID: 19224838]

[3]   Schütte K, Bornschein J, Malfertheiner P. Hepatocellular carcinoma--epidemiological trends and risk factors. Dig Dis 2009; 27(2): 80-92.
[http://dx.doi.org/10.1159/000218339] [PMID: 19546545]

[4]   Tseng TC, Liu CJ, Yang HC, Su TH, Wang CC, Chen CL, *et al.* High levels of hepatitis B surface antigen increase risk of hepatocellular carcinoma in patients with low HBV load. Gastroenterology 2012; 142(5): 1140-9.
[http://dx.doi.org/10.1053/j.gastro.2012.02.007]

[5]   Lui HF. Screening for hepatocellular carcinoma. Int J Hepatol 2011. 363151.
[http://dx.doi.org/10.4061/2011/363151]

[6]   Uchino K, Tateishi R, Shiina S, *et al.* Hepatocellular carcinoma with extrahepatic metastasis: clinical features and prognostic factors. Cancer 2011; 117(19): 4475-83.
        [http://dx.doi.org/10.1002/cncr.25960] [PMID: 21437884]

[7]   Gish RG, Finn RS, Marrero JA. Extending survival with the use of targeted therapy in the treatment of hepatocellular carcinoma. Gastroenterol Hepatol (N Y) 2013; 9(4) (Suppl. 2): 1-24.
        [PMID: 24872793]

[8]   Kinoshita A, Onoda H, Fushiya N, Koike K, Nishino H, Tajiri H. Staging systems for hepatocellular carcinoma: Current status and future perspectives. World J Hepatol 2015; 7(3): 406-24.
        [http://dx.doi.org/10.4254/wjh.v7.i3.406] [PMID: 25848467]

[9]   Subramaniam S, Kelley RK, Venook AP. A review of hepatocellular carcinoma (HCC) staging systems. Chin Clin Oncol 2013; 2(4): 33.
        [PMID: 25841912]

[10]   Perry JF, Charlton B, Koorey DJ, *et al.* Outcome of patients with hepatocellular carcinoma referred to a tertiary centre with availability of multiple treatment options including cadaveric liver transplantation. Liver Int 2007; 27(9): 1240-8.
        [PMID: 17919236]

[11]   Ng KK, Vauthey JN, Pawlik TM, *et al.* International Cooperative Study Group on Hepatocellular Carcinoma. Is hepatic resection for large or multinodular hepatocellular carcinoma justified? Results from a multi-institutional database. Ann Surg Oncol 2005; 12(5): 364-73.
        [http://dx.doi.org/10.1245/ASO.2005.06.004] [PMID: 15915370]

[12]   Yang T, Lin C, Zhai J, *et al.* Surgical resection for advanced hepatocellular carcinoma according to Barcelona Clinic Liver Cancer (BCLC) staging. J Cancer Res Clin Oncol 2012; 138(7): 1121-9.
        [http://dx.doi.org/10.1007/s00432-012-1188-0] [PMID: 22402598]

[13]   Roayaie S, Obeidat K, Sposito C, *et al.* Resection of hepatocellular cancer ≤2 cm: results from two Western centers. Hepatology 2013; 57(4): 1426-35.
        [http://dx.doi.org/10.1002/hep.25832] [PMID: 22576353]

[14]   Zhou HB, Li QM, Zhong ZR, *et al.* Level of hepatitis B surface antigen might serve as a new marker to predict hepatocellular carcinoma recurrence following curative resection in patients with low viral load. Am J Cancer Res 2015; 5(2): 756-71.
        [PMID: 25973313]

[15]   Xiao L, Xiang LJ, Li JW, Chen J, Fan YD, Zheng SG. Laparoscopic *versus* open liver resection for hepatocellular carcinoma in posterosuperior segments. Surg Endosc 2015; 29(10): 2994-3001.
        [http://dx.doi.org/10.1007/s00464-015-4214-x] [PMID: 25899815]

[16]   Li N, Wu YR, Wu B, Lu MQ. Surgical and oncologic outcomes following laparoscopic *versus* open liver resection for hepatocellular carcinoma: A meta-analysis. Hepatol Res 2012; 42(1): 51-9.
        [http://dx.doi.org/10.1111/j.1872-034X.2011.00890.x] [PMID: 21988222]

[17]   Mazzaferro V, Bhoori S, Sposito C, *et al.* Milan criteria in liver transplantation for hepatocellular carcinoma: an evidence-based analysis of 15 years of experience. Liver Transpl 2011; 17 (Suppl. 2): S44-57.
        [http://dx.doi.org/10.1002/lt.22365] [PMID: 21695773]

[18]   Vitale A, Morales RR, Zanus G, *et al.* Italian Liver Cancer group. Barcelona Clinic Liver Cancer staging and transplant survival benefit for patients with hepatocellular carcinoma: a multicentre, cohort study. Lancet Oncol 2011; 12(7): 654-62.
        [http://dx.doi.org/10.1016/S1470-2045(11)70144-9] [PMID: 21684210]

[19]   Gomaa AI, Waked I. Recent advances in multidisciplinary management of hepatocellular carcinoma. World J Hepatol 2015; 7(4): 673-87.
        [http://dx.doi.org/10.4254/wjh.v7.i4.673] [PMID: 25866604]

[20]   Pang TC, Lam VW. Surgical management of hepatocellular carcinoma. World J Hepatol 2015; 7(2):

245-52.
[http://dx.doi.org/10.4254/wjh.v7.i2.245] [PMID: 25729479]

[21]   Rahman A, Assifi MM, Pedroso FE, *et al.* Is resection equivalent to transplantation for early cirrhotic patients with hepatocellular carcinoma? A meta-analysis. J Gastrointest Surg 2012; 16(10): 1897-909.
[http://dx.doi.org/10.1007/s11605-012-1973-8] [PMID: 22836922]

[22]   Dhir M, Lyden ER, Smith LM, Are C. Comparison of outcomes of transplantation and resection in patients with early hepatocellular carcinoma: a meta-analysis. HPB (Oxford) 2012; 14(9): 635-45.
[http://dx.doi.org/10.1111/j.1477-2574.2012.00500.x] [PMID: 22882201]

[23]   Kaido T, Morita S, Tanaka S, *et al.* Long-term outcomes of hepatic resection *versus* living donor liver transplantation for hepatocellular carcinoma: a propensity score-matching study. Dis Markers 2015. 425926
[http://dx.doi.org/10.1155/2015/425926]

[24]   Lencioni R. Loco-regional treatment of hepatocellular carcinoma. Hepatology 2010; 52(2): 762-73.
[http://dx.doi.org/10.1002/hep.23725] [PMID: 20564355]

[25]   Huang GT, Lee PH, Tsang YM, *et al.* Percutaneous ethanol injection *versus* surgical resection for the treatment of small hepatocellular carcinoma: a prospective study. Ann Surg 2005; 242(1): 36-42.
[http://dx.doi.org/10.1097/01.sla.0000167925.90380.fe] [PMID: 15973099]

[26]   Lencioni R, Cioni D, Crocetti L, Bartolozzi C. Percutaneous ablation of hepatocellular carcinoma: state-of-the-art. Liver Transpl 2004; 10(2) (Suppl. 1): S91-7.
[http://dx.doi.org/10.1002/lt.20043] [PMID: 14762847]

[27]   Liang HL, Yang CF, Pan HB, *et al.* Small hepatocellular carcinoma: safety and efficacy of single high-dose percutaneous acetic acid injection for treatment. Radiology 2000; 214(3): 769-74.
[http://dx.doi.org/10.1148/radiology.214.3.r00mr06769] [PMID: 10715044]

[28]   Germani G, Pleguezuelo M, Gurusamy K, Meyer T, Isgrò G, Burroughs AK. Clinical outcomes of radiofrequency ablation, percutaneous alcohol and acetic acid injection for hepatocelullar carcinoma: a meta-analysis. J Hepatol 2010; 52(3): 380-8.
[http://dx.doi.org/10.1016/j.jhep.2009.12.004] [PMID: 20149473]

[29]   Lin SM, Lin CJ, Lin CC, Hsu CW, Chen YC. Radiofrequency ablation improves prognosis compared with ethanol injection for hepatocellular carcinoma < or =4 cm. Gastroenterology 2004; 127(6): 1714-23.
[http://dx.doi.org/10.1053/j.gastro.2004.09.003] [PMID: 15578509]

[30]   Lin SM, Lin CJ, Lin CC, Hsu CW, Chen YC. Randomised controlled trial comparing percutaneous radiofrequency thermal ablation, percutaneous ethanol injection, and percutaneous acetic acid injection to treat hepatocellular carcinoma of 3 cm or less. Gut 2005; 54(8): 1151-6.
[http://dx.doi.org/10.1136/gut.2004.045203] [PMID: 16009687]

[31]   Zhang L, Ge NL, Chen Y, *et al.* Long-term outcomes and prognostic analysis of radiofrequency ablation for small hepatocellular carcinoma: 10-year follow-up in Chinese patients. Med Oncol 2015; 32(3): 77.
[http://dx.doi.org/10.1007/s12032-015-0532-z] [PMID: 25698535]

[32]   Chen X, Chen Y, Li Q, Ma D, Shen B, Peng C. Radiofrequency ablation *versus* surgical resection for intrahepatic hepatocellular carcinoma recurrence: a meta-analysis. J Surg Res 2015; 195(1): 166-74.
[http://dx.doi.org/10.1016/j.jss.2015.01.042] [PMID: 25724768]

[33]   Wang JH, Wang CC, Hung CH, Chen CL, Lu SN. Survival comparison between surgical resection and radiofrequency ablation for patients in BCLC very early/early stage hepatocellular carcinoma. J Hepatol 2012; 56(2): 412-8.
[http://dx.doi.org/10.1016/j.jhep.2011.05.020] [PMID: 21756858]

[34]   Schramm W, Yang D, Wood BJ, Rattay F, Haemmerich D. Contribution of direct heating, thermal conduction and perfusion during radiofrequency and microwave ablation. Open Biomed Eng J 2007;

1: 47-52.
[http://dx.doi.org/10.2174/1874120700701010047] [PMID: 19662127]

[35]   Ding J, Jing X, Liu J, *et al.* Comparison of two different thermal techniques for the treatment of hepatocellular carcinoma. Eur J Radiol 2013; 82(9): 1379-84.
[http://dx.doi.org/10.1016/j.ejrad.2013.04.025] [PMID: 23726122]

[36]   Zhang L, Wang N, Shen Q, Cheng W, Qian GJ. Therapeutic efficacy of percutaneous radiofrequency ablation *versus* microwave ablation for hepatocellular carcinoma. PLoS One 2013; 8(10): e76119.
[http://dx.doi.org/10.1371/journal.pone.0076119] [PMID: 24146824]

[37]   Pacella CM, Bizzarri G, Francica G, *et al.* Percutaneous laser ablation in the treatment of hepatocellular carcinoma with small tumors: analysis of factors affecting the achievement of tumor necrosis. J Vasc Interv Radiol 2005; 16(11): 1447-57.
[http://dx.doi.org/10.1097/01.RVI.90000172121.82299.38] [PMID: 16319150]

[38]   Ferrari FS, Megliola A, Scorzelli A, *et al.* Treatment of small HCC through radiofrequency ablation and laser ablation. Comparison of techniques and long-term results. Radiol Med (Torino) 2007; 112(3): 377-93.
[http://dx.doi.org/10.1007/s11547-007-0148-2] [PMID: 17447018]

[39]   Rong G, Bai W, Dong Z, *et al.* Cryotherapy for cirrhosis-based hepatocellular carcinoma: a single center experience from 1595 treated cases. Front Med 2015; 9(1): 63-71.
[http://dx.doi.org/10.1007/s11684-014-0342-2] [PMID: 25001101]

[40]   Rong G, Bai W, Dong Z, *et al.* Long-term outcomes of percutaneous cryoablation for patients with hepatocellular carcinoma within Milan criteria. PLoS One 2015; 10(4): e0123065.
[http://dx.doi.org/10.1371/journal.pone.0123065] [PMID: 25849963]

[41]   Ei S, Hibi T, Tanabe M, *et al.* Cryoablation provides superior local control of primary hepatocellular carcinomas of >2 cm compared with radiofrequency ablation and microwave coagulation therapy: an underestimated tool in the toolbox. Ann Surg Oncol 2015; 22(4): 1294-300.
[http://dx.doi.org/10.1245/s10434-014-4114-7] [PMID: 25287439]

[42]   Wang C, Wang H, Yang W, *et al.* Multicenter randomized controlled trial of percutaneous cryoablation *versus* radiofrequency ablation in hepatocellular carcinoma. Hepatology 2015; 61(5): 1579-90.
[http://dx.doi.org/10.1002/hep.27548] [PMID: 25284802]

[43]   Oliveri RS, Wetterslev J, Gluud C. Transarterial (chemo)embolisation for unresectable hepatocellular carcinoma. Cochrane Database Syst Rev 2011; (3): CD004787.
[PMID: 21412886]

[44]   Lo CM, Ngan H, Tso WK, *et al.* Randomized controlled trial of transarterial lipiodol chemoembolization for unresectable hepatocellular carcinoma. Hepatology 2002; 35(5): 1164-71.
[http://dx.doi.org/10.1053/jhep.2002.33156] [PMID: 11981766]

[45]   Doffoël M, Bonnetain F, Bouché O, *et al.* Fédération Francophone de Cancérologie Digestive. Multicentre randomised phase III trial comparing Tamoxifen alone or with Transarterial Lipiodol Chemoembolisation for unresectable hepatocellular carcinoma in cirrhotic patients (Fédération Francophone de Cancérologie Digestive 9402). Eur J Cancer 2008; 44(4): 528-38.
[http://dx.doi.org/10.1016/j.ejca.2008.01.004] [PMID: 18242076]

[46]   Takayasu K, Arii S, Ikai I, *et al.* Liver Cancer Study Group of Japan. Prospective cohort study of transarterial chemoembolization for unresectable hepatocellular carcinoma in 8510 patients. Gastroenterology 2006; 131(2): 461-9.
[http://dx.doi.org/10.1053/j.gastro.2006.05.021] [PMID: 16890600]

[47]   Paul SB, Gamanagatti S, Sreenivas V, *et al.* Trans-arterial chemoembolization (TACE) in patients with unresectable Hepatocellular carcinoma: Experience from a tertiary care centre in India. Indian J Radiol Imaging 2011; 21(2): 113-20.
[http://dx.doi.org/10.4103/0971-3026.82294] [PMID: 21799594]

[48]　Okusaka T, Kasugai H, Shioyama Y, *et al.* Transarterial chemotherapy alone *versus* transarterial chemoembolization for hepatocellular carcinoma: a randomized phase III trial. J Hepatol 2009; 51(6): 1030-6.
[http://dx.doi.org/10.1016/j.jhep.2009.09.004] [PMID: 19864035]

[49]　Leung DA, Goin JE, Sickles C, Raskay BJ, Soulen MC. Determinants of postembolization syndrome after hepatic chemoembolization. J Vasc Interv Radiol 2001; 12(3): 321-6.
[http://dx.doi.org/10.1016/S1051-0443(07)61911-3] [PMID: 11287509]

[50]　Salem R, Lewandowski RJ, Kulik L, *et al.* Radioembolization results in longer time-to-progression and reduced toxicity compared with chemoembolization in patients with hepatocellular carcinoma. Gastroenterology 2011; 140(2): 497-507.e2.
[http://dx.doi.org/10.1053/j.gastro.2010.10.049] [PMID: 21044630]

[51]　Carr BI, Kondragunta V, Buch SC, Branch RA. Therapeutic equivalence in survival for hepatic arterial chemoembolization and yttrium 90 microsphere treatments in unresectable hepatocellular carcinoma: a two-cohort study. Cancer 2010; 116(5): 1305-14.
[http://dx.doi.org/10.1002/cncr.24884] [PMID: 20066715]

[52]　Ozkan ZG, Poyanli A, Ucar A, *et al.* Favorable survival time provided with radioembolization in hepatocellular carcinoma patients with and without portal vein thrombosis. Cancer Biother Radiopharm 2015; 30(3): 132-8.
[http://dx.doi.org/10.1089/cbr.2014.1748] [PMID: 25760644]

[53]　European Association For The Study Of The Liver; European Organisation For Research And Treatment Of Cancer. EASL-EORTC clinical practice guidelines: management of hepatocellular carcinoma. J Hepatol 2012; 56(4): 908-43.
[http://dx.doi.org/10.1016/j.jhep.2011.12.001] [PMID: 22424438]

[54]　Yeo W, Mok TS, Zee B, *et al.* A randomized phase III study of doxorubicin *versus* cisplatin/interferon alpha-2b/doxorubicin/fluorouracil (PIAF) combination chemotherapy for unresectable hepatocellular carcinoma. J Natl Cancer Inst 2005; 97(20): 1532-8.
[http://dx.doi.org/10.1093/jnci/dji315] [PMID: 16234567]

[55]　Sukowati CH, Rosso N, Pascut D, *et al.* Gene and functional up-regulation of the BCRP/ABCG2 transporter in hepatocellular carcinoma. BMC Gastroenterol 2012; 12: 160.
[http://dx.doi.org/10.1186/1471-230X-12-160] [PMID: 23153066]

[56]　Cao LQ, Wang XL, Wang Q, *et al.* Rosiglitazone sensitizes hepatocellular carcinoma cell lines to 5-fluorouracil antitumor activity through activation of the PPARgamma signaling pathway. Acta Pharmacol Sin 2009; 30(9): 1316-22.
[http://dx.doi.org/10.1038/aps.2009.119] [PMID: 19684609]

[57]　Gish RG, Porta C, Lazar L, *et al.* Phase III randomized controlled trial comparing the survival of patients with unresectable hepatocellular carcinoma treated with nolatrexed or doxorubicin. J Clin Oncol 2007; 25(21): 3069-75.
[http://dx.doi.org/10.1200/JCO.2006.08.4046] [PMID: 17634485]

[58]　Qin S, Bai Y, Lim HY, *et al.* Randomized, multicenter, open-label study of oxaliplatin plus fluorouracil/leucovorin *versus* doxorubicin as palliative chemotherapy in patients with advanced hepatocellular carcinoma from Asia. J Clin Oncol 2013; 31(28): 3501-8.
[http://dx.doi.org/10.1200/JCO.2012.44.5643] [PMID: 23980077]

[59]　Llovet JM, Ricci S, Mazzaferro V, *et al.* SHARP Investigators Study Group. Sorafenib in advanced hepatocellular carcinoma. N Engl J Med 2008; 359(4): 378-90.
[http://dx.doi.org/10.1056/NEJMoa0708857] [PMID: 18650514]

[60]　Cheng AL, Kang YK, Chen Z, *et al.* Efficacy and safety of sorafenib in patients in the Asia-Pacific region with advanced hepatocellular carcinoma: a phase III randomised, double-blind, placebo-controlled trial. Lancet Oncol 2009; 10(1): 25-34.
[http://dx.doi.org/10.1016/S1470-2045(08)70285-7] [PMID: 19095497]

[61]   Cheng AL, Kang YK, Lin DY, *et al.* Sunitinib *versus* sorafenib in advanced hepatocellular cancer: results of a randomized phase III trial. J Clin Oncol 2013; 31(32): 4067-75.
[http://dx.doi.org/10.1200/JCO.2012.45.8372] [PMID: 24081937]

[62]   Llovet JM, Decaens T, Raoul JL, *et al.* Brivanib in patients with advanced hepatocellular carcinoma who were intolerant to sorafenib or for whom sorafenib failed: results from the randomized phase III BRISK-PS study. J Clin Oncol 2013; 31(28): 3509-16.
[http://dx.doi.org/10.1200/JCO.2012.47.3009] [PMID: 23980090]

[63]   Johnson PJ, Qin S, Park JW, *et al.* Brivanib *versus* sorafenib as first-line therapy in patients with unresectable, advanced hepatocellular carcinoma: results from the randomized phase III BRISK-FL study. J Clin Oncol 2013; 31(28): 3517-24.
[http://dx.doi.org/10.1200/JCO.2012.48.4410] [PMID: 23980084]

[64]   Cainap C, Qin S, Huang WT, *et al.* Linifanib *versus* Sorafenib in patients with advanced hepatocellular carcinoma: results of a randomized phase III trial. J Clin Oncol 2015; 33(2): 172-9.
[http://dx.doi.org/10.1200/JCO.2013.54.3298] [PMID: 25488963]

[65]   Zhu AX, Kudo M, Assenat E, *et al.* Effect of everolimus on survival in advanced hepatocellular carcinoma after failure of sorafenib: the EVOLVE-1 randomized clinical trial. JAMA 2014; 312(1): 57-67.
[http://dx.doi.org/10.1001/jama.2014.7189] [PMID: 25058218]

[66]   Hollebecque A, Malka D, Ferté C, Ducreux M, Boige V. Systemic treatment of advanced hepatocellular carcinoma: from disillusions to new horizons. Eur J Cancer 2015; 51(3): 327-39.
[http://dx.doi.org/10.1016/j.ejca.2014.12.005] [PMID: 25559615]

[67]   Printz C. Clinical trials of note. Sorafenib as adjuvant treatment in the prevention of disease recurrence in patients with hepatocellular carcinoma (HCC) (STORM). Cancer 2009; 115(20): 4646.
[http://dx.doi.org/10.1002/cncr.24673] [PMID: 19806596]

[68]   Pawlik TM, Reyes DK, Cosgrove D, Kamel IR, Bhagat N, Geschwind JF. Phase II trial of sorafenib combined with concurrent transarterial chemoembolization with drug-eluting beads for hepatocellular carcinoma. J Clin Oncol 2011; 29(30): 3960-7.
[http://dx.doi.org/10.1200/JCO.2011.37.1021] [PMID: 21911714]

[69]   Park JW, Koh YH, Kim HB, *et al.* Phase II study of concurrent transarterial chemoembolization and sorafenib in patients with unresectable hepatocellular carcinoma. J Hepatol 2012; 56(6): 1336-42.
[http://dx.doi.org/10.1016/j.jhep.2012.01.006] [PMID: 22314421]

[70]   Sansonno D, Lauletta G, Russi S, Conteduca V, Sansonno L, Dammacco F. Transarterial chemoembolization plus sorafenib: a sequential therapeutic scheme for HCV-related intermediate-stage hepatocellular carcinoma: a randomized clinical trial. Oncologist 2012; 17(3): 359-66.
[http://dx.doi.org/10.1634/theoncologist.2011-0313] [PMID: 22334456]

[71]   Kudo M, Imanaka K, Chida N, *et al.* Phase III study of sorafenib after transarterial chemoembolisation in Japanese and Korean patients with unresectable hepatocellular carcinoma. Eur J Cancer 2011; 47(14): 2117-27.
[http://dx.doi.org/10.1016/j.ejca.2011.05.007] [PMID: 21664811]

[72]   Hu H, Duan Z, Long X, *et al.* Sorafenib combined with transarterial chemoembolization *versus* transarterial chemoembolization alone for advanced-stage hepatocellular carcinoma: a propensity score matching study. PLoS One 2014; 9(5): e96620.
[http://dx.doi.org/10.1371/journal.pone.0096620] [PMID: 24817002]

[73]   Faivre S, Raymond E, Boucher E, *et al.* Safety and efficacy of sunitinib in patients with advanced hepatocellular carcinoma: an open-label, multicentre, phase II study. Lancet Oncol 2009; 10(8): 794-800.
[http://dx.doi.org/10.1016/S1470-2045(09)70171-8] [PMID: 19586800]

[74]   Barone C, Basso M, Biolato M, *et al.* A phase II study of sunitinib in advanced hepatocellular

carcinoma. Dig Liver Dis 2013; 45(8): 692-8.
[http://dx.doi.org/10.1016/j.dld.2013.01.002] [PMID: 23410734]

[75]   Koeberle D, Montemurro M, Samaras P, *et al.* Continuous Sunitinib treatment in patients with advanced hepatocellular carcinoma: a Swiss Group for Clinical Cancer Research (SAKK) and Swiss Association for the Study of the Liver (SASL) multicenter phase II trial (SAKK 77/06). Oncologist 2010; 15(3): 285-92.
[http://dx.doi.org/10.1634/theoncologist.2009-0316] [PMID: 20203173]

[76]   Huynh H, Ngo VC, Fargnoli J, *et al.* Brivanib alaninate, a dual inhibitor of vascular endothelial growth factor receptor and fibroblast growth factor receptor tyrosine kinases, induces growth inhibition in mouse models of human hepatocellular carcinoma. Clin Cancer Res 2008; 14(19): 6146-53.
[http://dx.doi.org/10.1158/1078-0432.CCR-08-0509] [PMID: 18829493]

[77]   Kudo M, Han G, Finn RS, *et al.* Brivanib as adjuvant therapy to transarterial chemoembolization in patients with hepatocellular carcinoma: A randomized phase III trial. Hepatology 2014; 60(5): 1697-707.
[http://dx.doi.org/10.1002/hep.27290] [PMID: 24996197]

[78]   Kanai F, Yoshida H, Tateishi R, *et al.* A phase I/II trial of the oral antiangiogenic agent TSU-68 in patients with advanced hepatocellular carcinoma. Cancer Chemother Pharmacol 2011; 67(2): 315-24.
[http://dx.doi.org/10.1007/s00280-010-1320-2] [PMID: 20390419]

[79]   Inaba Y, Kanai F, Aramaki T, *et al.* A randomised phase II study of TSU-68 in patients with hepatocellular carcinoma treated by transarterial chemoembolisation. Eur J Cancer 2013; 49(13): 2832-40.
[http://dx.doi.org/10.1016/j.ejca.2013.05.011] [PMID: 23764238]

[80]   Alberts SR, Fitch TR, Kim GP, *et al.* Cediranib (AZD2171) in patients with advanced hepatocellular carcinoma: a phase II North Central Cancer Treatment Group Clinical Trial. Am J Clin Oncol 2012; 35(4): 329-33.
[http://dx.doi.org/10.1097/COC.0b013e3182118cdf] [PMID: 21422991]

[81]   Zhu AX, Ancukiewicz M, Supko JG, *et al.* Efficacy, safety, pharmacokinetics, and biomarkers of cediranib monotherapy in advanced hepatocellular carcinoma: a phase II study. Clin Cancer Res 2013; 19(6): 1557-66.
[http://dx.doi.org/10.1158/1078-0432.CCR-12-3041] [PMID: 23362324]

[82]   Kondo S, Ojima H, Tsuda H, *et al.* Clinical impact of c-Met expression and its gene amplification in hepatocellular carcinoma. Int J Clin Oncol 2013; 18(2): 207-13.
[http://dx.doi.org/10.1007/s10147-011-0361-9] [PMID: 22218908]

[83]   Santoro A, Rimassa L, Borbath I, *et al.* Tivantinib for second-line treatment of advanced hepatocellular carcinoma: a randomised, placebo-controlled phase 2 study. Lancet Oncol 2013; 14(1): 55-63.
[http://dx.doi.org/10.1016/S1470-2045(12)70490-4] [PMID: 23182627]

[84]   Xiang Q, Chen W, Ren M, *et al.* Cabozantinib suppresses tumor growth and metastasis in hepatocellular carcinoma by a dual blockade of VEGFR2 and MET. Clin Cancer Res 2014; 20(11): 2959-70.
[http://dx.doi.org/10.1158/1078-0432.CCR-13-2620] [PMID: 24700742]

[85]   Sahin F, Kannangai R, Adegbola O, Wang J, Su G, Torbenson M. mTOR and P70 S6 kinase expression in primary liver neoplasms. Clin Cancer Res 2004; 10(24): 8421-5.
[http://dx.doi.org/10.1158/1078-0432.CCR-04-0941] [PMID: 15623621]

[86]   Villanueva A, Chiang DY, Newell P, *et al.* Pivotal role of mTOR signaling in hepatocellular carcinoma. Gastroenterology 2008; 135(6): 1-11.
[http://dx.doi.org/10.1053/j.gastro.2008.08.008]

[87]   Huynh H, Chow KH, Soo KC, *et al.* RAD001 (everolimus) inhibits tumour growth in xenograft models of human hepatocellular carcinoma. J Cell Mol Med 2009; 13(7): 1371-80.

[http://dx.doi.org/10.1111/j.1582-4934.2008.00364.x] [PMID: 18466352]

[88] Zhu AX, Abrams TA, Miksad R, *et al.* Phase 1/2 study of everolimus in advanced hepatocellular carcinoma. Cancer 2011; 117(22): 5094-102.
[http://dx.doi.org/10.1002/cncr.26165] [PMID: 21538343]

[89] Huynh H, Hao HX, Chan SL, *et al.* Loss of tuberous sclerosis complex 2 (TSC2) is frequent in hepatocellular carcinoma and predicts response to mTORC1 inhibitor everolimus. Mol Cancer Ther 2015; 14(5): 1224-35.
[http://dx.doi.org/10.1158/1535-7163.MCT-14-0768] [PMID: 25724664]

[90] Schnitzbauer AA, Zuelke C, Graeb C, *et al.* A prospective randomised, open-labeled, trial comparing sirolimus-containing *versus* mTOR-inhibitor-free immunosuppression in patients undergoing liver transplantation for hepatocellular carcinoma. BMC Cancer 2010; 10: 190.
[http://dx.doi.org/10.1186/1471-2407-10-190] [PMID: 20459775]

[91] Pardoll DM. The blockade of immune checkpoints in cancer immunotherapy. Nat Rev Cancer 2012; 12(4): 252-64.
[http://dx.doi.org/10.1038/nrc3239] [PMID: 22437870]

[92] Hodi FS, O'Day SJ, McDermott DF, *et al.* Improved survival with ipilimumab in patients with metastatic melanoma. N Engl J Med 2010; 363(8): 711-23.
[http://dx.doi.org/10.1056/NEJMoa1003466] [PMID: 20525992]

[93] Kuang DM, Zhao Q, Peng C, *et al.* Activated monocytes in peritumoral stroma of hepatocellular carcinoma foster immune privilege and disease progression through PD-L1. J Exp Med 2009; 206(6): 1327-37.
[http://dx.doi.org/10.1084/jem.20082173] [PMID: 19451266]

[94] Chen CJ, Yang HI, Su J, *et al.* REVEAL-HBV Study Group. Risk of hepatocellular carcinoma across a biological gradient of serum hepatitis B virus DNA level. JAMA 2006; 295(1): 65-73.
[http://dx.doi.org/10.1001/jama.295.1.65] [PMID: 16391218]

[95] Iloeje UH, Yang HI, Su J, Jen CL, You SL, Chen CJ. Predicting cirrhosis risk based on the level of circulating hepatitis B viral load. Gastroenterology 2006; 130(3): 678-86.
[http://dx.doi.org/10.1053/j.gastro.2005.11.016] [PMID: 16530509]

[96] Yu MW, Yeh SH, Chen PJ, *et al.* Hepatitis B virus genotype and DNA level and hepatocellular carcinoma: a prospective study in men. J Natl Cancer Inst 2005; 97(4): 265-72.
[http://dx.doi.org/10.1093/jnci/dji043] [PMID: 15713961]

[97] Yang HI, Lu SN, Liaw YF, *et al.* Taiwan Community-Based Cancer Screening Project Group. Hepatitis B e antigen and the risk of hepatocellular carcinoma. N Engl J Med 2002; 347(3): 168-74.
[http://dx.doi.org/10.1056/NEJMoa013215] [PMID: 12124405]

[98] An HJ, Jang JW, Bae SH, *et al.* Sustained low hepatitis B viral load predicts good outcome after curative resection in patients with hepatocellular carcinoma. J Gastroenterol Hepatol 2010; 25(12): 1876-82.
[http://dx.doi.org/10.1111/j.1440-1746.2010.06416.x] [PMID: 21092000]

[99] Huang G, Lai EC, Lau WY, *et al.* Posthepatectomy HBV reactivation in hepatitis B-related hepatocellular carcinoma influences postoperative survival in patients with preoperative low HBV-DNA levels. Ann Surg 2013; 257(3): 490-505.
[http://dx.doi.org/10.1097/SLA.0b013e318262b218] [PMID: 22868358]

[100] Someya T, Ikeda K, Saitoh S, *et al.* Interferon lowers tumor recurrence rate after surgical resection or ablation of hepatocellular carcinoma: a pilot study of patients with hepatitis B virus-related cirrhosis. J Gastroenterol 2006; 41(12): 1206-13.
[http://dx.doi.org/10.1007/s00535-006-1912-0] [PMID: 17287900]

[101] Lo CM, Liu CL, Chan SC, *et al.* A randomized, controlled trial of postoperative adjuvant interferon therapy after resection of hepatocellular carcinoma. Ann Surg 2007; 245(6): 831-42.

[http://dx.doi.org/10.1097/01.sla.0000245829.00977.45] [PMID: 17522506]

[102] Sun HC, Tang ZY, Wang L, *et al.* Postoperative interferon alpha treatment postponed recurrence and improved overall survival in patients after curative resection of HBV-related hepatocellular carcinoma: a randomized clinical trial. J Cancer Res Clin Oncol 2006; 132(7): 458-65.
[http://dx.doi.org/10.1007/s00432-006-0091-y] [PMID: 16557381]

[103] Chen LT, Chen MF, Li LA, *et al.* Disease Committee of Adjuvant Therapy for Postoperative Hepatocellular Carcinoma, Taiwan Cooperative Oncology Group, National Health Research Institutes, Zhunan, Taiwan. Long-term results of a randomized, observation-controlled, phase III trial of adjuvant interferon Alfa-2b in hepatocellular carcinoma after curative resection. Ann Surg 2012; 255(1): 8-17.
[http://dx.doi.org/10.1097/SLA.0b013e3182363ff9] [PMID: 22104564]

[104] Liaw YF, Sung JJ, Chow WC, *et al.* Cirrhosis Asian Lamivudine Multicentre Study Group. Lamivudine for patients with chronic hepatitis B and advanced liver disease. N Engl J Med 2004; 351(15): 1521-31.
[http://dx.doi.org/10.1056/NEJMoa033364] [PMID: 15470215]

[105] Kuzuya T, Katano Y, Kumada T, *et al.* Efficacy of antiviral therapy with lamivudine after initial treatment for hepatitis B virus-related hepatocellular carcinoma. J Gastroenterol Hepatol 2007; 22(11): 1929-35.
[http://dx.doi.org/10.1111/j.1440-1746.2006.04707.x] [PMID: 17914972]

[106] Chuma M, Hige S, Kamiyama T, *et al.* The influence of hepatitis B DNA level and antiviral therapy on recurrence after initial curative treatment in patients with hepatocellular carcinoma. J Gastroenterol 2009; 44(9): 991-9.
[http://dx.doi.org/10.1007/s00535-009-0093-z] [PMID: 19554391]

[107] Yoshida H, Yoshida H, Goto E, *et al.* Safety and efficacy of lamivudine after radiofrequency ablation in patients with hepatitis B virus-related hepatocellular carcinoma. Hepatol Int 2008; 2(1): 89-94.
[http://dx.doi.org/10.1007/s12072-007-9020-7] [PMID: 19669283]

[108] Yin J, Li N, Han Y, *et al.* Effect of antiviral treatment with nucleotide/nucleoside analogs on postoperative prognosis of hepatitis B virus-related hepatocellular carcinoma: a two-stage longitudinal clinical study. J Clin Oncol 2013; 31(29): 3647-55.
[http://dx.doi.org/10.1200/JCO.2012.48.5896] [PMID: 24002499]

[109] Nishikawa H, Nishijima N, Arimoto A, *et al.* Effect of nucleoside analog use in patients with hepatitis B virus-related hepatocellular carcinoma. Hepatol Res 2014; 44(6): 608-20.
[http://dx.doi.org/10.1111/hepr.12169] [PMID: 23701455]

[110] Wu CY, Chen YJ, Ho HJ, *et al.* Association between nucleoside analogues and risk of hepatitis B virus–related hepatocellular carcinoma recurrence following liver resection. JAMA 2012; 308(18): 1906-14.
[http://dx.doi.org/10.1001/2012.jama.11975] [PMID: 23162861]

[111] Lai CL, Gane E, Liaw YF, *et al.* Globe Study Group. Telbivudine *versus* lamivudine in patients with chronic hepatitis B. N Engl J Med 2007; 357(25): 2576-88.
[http://dx.doi.org/10.1056/NEJMoa066422] [PMID: 18094378]

[112] Chang TT, Gish RG, de Man R, *et al.* BEHoLD AI463022 Study Group. A comparison of entecavir and lamivudine for HBeAg-positive chronic hepatitis B. N Engl J Med 2006; 354(10): 1001-10.
[http://dx.doi.org/10.1056/NEJMoa051285] [PMID: 16525137]

[113] Lai CL, Rosmawati M, Lao J, *et al.* Entecavir is superior to lamivudine in reducing hepatitis B virus DNA in patients with chronic hepatitis B infection. Gastroenterology 2002; 123(6): 1831-8.
[http://dx.doi.org/10.1053/gast.2002.37058] [PMID: 12454840]

[114] Sung JJ, Lai JY, Zeuzem S, *et al.* Lamivudine compared with lamivudine and adefovir dipivoxil for the treatment of HBeAg-positive chronic hepatitis B. J Hepatol 2008; 48(5): 728-35.
[http://dx.doi.org/10.1016/j.jhep.2007.12.026] [PMID: 18329126]

[115] Lai CL, Leung N, Teo EK, *et al.* Telbivudine Phase II Investigator Group. A 1-year trial of telbivudine, lamivudine, and the combination in patients with hepatitis B e antigen-positive chronic hepatitis B. Gastroenterology 2005; 129(2): 528-36.
[http://dx.doi.org/10.1016/j.gastro.2005.05.053] [PMID: 16083710]

[116] Lai CL, Dienstag J, Schiff E, *et al.* Prevalence and clinical correlates of YMDD variants during lamivudine therapy for patients with chronic hepatitis B. Clin Infect Dis 2003; 36(6): 687-96.
[http://dx.doi.org/10.1086/368083] [PMID: 12627352]

[117] Pearlman BL, Traub N. Sustained virologic response to antiviral therapy for chronic hepatitis C virus infection: a cure and so much more. Clin Infect Dis 2011; 52(7): 889-900.
[http://dx.doi.org/10.1093/cid/cir076] [PMID: 21427396]

[118] Jazwinski AB, Muir AJ. Direct-acting antiviral medications for chronic hepatitis C virus infection. Gastroenterol Hepatol (N Y) 2011; 7(3): 154-62.
[PMID: 21528041]

[119] Hsu YC, Wu CY, Lin JT. Hepatitis C virus infection, antiviral therapy, and risk of hepatocellular carcinoma. Semin Oncol 2015; 42(2): 329-38.
[http://dx.doi.org/10.1053/j.seminoncol.2014.12.023] [PMID: 25843737]

[120] Mir HM, Birerdinc A, Younossi ZM. Monoclonal and polyclonal antibodies against the HCV envelope proteins. Clin Liver Dis 2009; 13(3): 477-86.
[http://dx.doi.org/10.1016/j.cld.2009.05.011] [PMID: 19628163]

[121] Pawlotsky JM, Chevaliez S, McHutchison JG. The hepatitis C virus life cycle as a target for new antiviral therapies. Gastroenterology 2007; 132(5): 1979-98.
[http://dx.doi.org/10.1053/j.gastro.2007.03.116] [PMID: 17484890]

[122] Zhang YQ, Guo JS. Antiviral therapies for hepatitis B virus-related hepatocellular carcinoma. World J Gastroenterol 2015; 21(13): 3860-6.
[http://dx.doi.org/10.3748/wjg.v21.i13.3860] [PMID: 25852270]

[123] Kwo PY, Lawitz EJ, McCone J, *et al.* SPRINT-1 investigators. Efficacy of boceprevir, an NS3 protease inhibitor, in combination with peginterferon alfa-2b and ribavirin in treatment-naive patients with genotype 1 hepatitis C infection (SPRINT-1): an open-label, randomised, multicentre phase 2 trial. Lancet 2010; 376(9742): 705-16.
[http://dx.doi.org/10.1016/S0140-6736(10)60934-8] [PMID: 20692693]

[124] Bacon BR, Gordon SC, Lawitz E, *et al.* HCV RESPOND-2 Investigators. Boceprevir for previously treated chronic HCV genotype 1 infection. N Engl J Med 2011; 364(13): 1207-17.
[http://dx.doi.org/10.1056/NEJMoa1009482] [PMID: 21449784]

[125] Jacobson IM, McHutchison JG, Dusheiko G, *et al.* ADVANCE Study Team. Telaprevir for previously untreated chronic hepatitis C virus infection. N Engl J Med 2011; 364(25): 2405-16.
[http://dx.doi.org/10.1056/NEJMoa1012912] [PMID: 21696307]

[126] Zeuzem S, Andreone P, Pol S, *et al.* REALIZE Study Team. Telaprevir for retreatment of HCV infection. N Engl J Med 2011; 364(25): 2417-28.
[http://dx.doi.org/10.1056/NEJMoa1013086] [PMID: 21696308]

[127] Nagpal N, Goyal S, Wahi D, *et al.* Molecular principles behind Boceprevir resistance due to mutations in hepatitis C NS3/4A protease. Gene 2015; 570(1): 115-21.
[http://dx.doi.org/10.1016/j.gene.2015.06.008] [PMID: 26055089]

[128] Kieffer TL, Sarrazin C, Miller JS, *et al.* Telaprevir and pegylated interferon-alpha-2a inhibit wild-type and resistant genotype 1 hepatitis C virus replication in patients. Hepatology 2007; 46(3): 631-9.
[http://dx.doi.org/10.1002/hep.21781] [PMID: 17680654]

[129] Asselah T. Sofosbuvir for the treatment of hepatitis C virus. Expert Opin Pharmacother 2014; 15(1): 121-30.
[http://dx.doi.org/10.1517/14656566.2014.857656] [PMID: 24289735]

[130] Lawitz E, Mangia A, Wyles D, *et al.* Sofosbuvir for previously untreated chronic hepatitis C infection. N Engl J Med 2013; 368(20): 1878-87.
[http://dx.doi.org/10.1056/NEJMoa1214853] [PMID: 23607594]

[131] Jacobson IM, Gordon SC, Kowdley KV, *et al.* POSITRON Study; FUSION Study. Sofosbuvir for hepatitis C genotype 2 or 3 in patients without treatment options. N Engl J Med 2013; 368(20): 1867-77.
[http://dx.doi.org/10.1056/NEJMoa1214854] [PMID: 23607593]

[132] Sims KD, Lemm J, Eley T, *et al.* Randomized, placebo-controlled, single-ascending-dose study of BMS-791325, a hepatitis C virus (HCV) NS5B polymerase inhibitor, in HCV genotype 1 infection. Antimicrob Agents Chemother 2014; 58(6): 3496-503.
[http://dx.doi.org/10.1128/AAC.02579-13] [PMID: 24733462]

[133] Conti F, Buonfiglioli F, Scuteri A, *et al.* Early occurrence and recurrence of hepatocellular carcinoma in HCV-related cirrhosis treated with direct-acting antivirals. J Hepatol 2016; 65(4): 727-33.
[http://dx.doi.org/10.1016/j.jhep.2016.06.015] [PMID: 27349488]

[134] Reig M, Mariño Z, Perelló C, *et al.* Unexpected high rate of early tumor recurrence in patients with HCV-related HCC undergoing interferon-free therapy. J Hepatol 2016; S0168-8278(16)30113-1.
[PMID: 27084592]

CHAPTER 5

Recent Development (from 2013 to 2015) of Gold-Based Compounds as Potential Anti-Cancer Drug Candidates

Raymond Wai-Yin Sun[123]*, **Chunxia Chen[2]**, **Man-Kin Tse[2]**, **Chih-Chiang Chen[2]** and **Albert S.-C. Chan[2]**

[1] *Department of Chemistry, Shantou University, 243 Daxue Road, Shantou, Guangdong 515063, P.R. China*

[2] *Guangzhou Lee & Man Technology Company Limited, Nansha, Guangzhou, Guangdong, P.R. China*

[3] *Department of Chemistry, The University of Hong Kong, Pokfulam Road, Hong Kong*

Abstract: Cisplatin (Fig. **1**) is a platinum(II) compound which contains two chlorido and two ammino ligands. In 1965 the biological activity of this compound was serendipitously discovered by Rosenberg *et al.* At present, this platinum(II) compound remains one of the effective chemotherapeutic agents for the treatment of various cancers in clinic [1]. The clinical success of this platinum compound has subsequently prompted the studies to identify other new metal-based therapeutic agents. As compared to organic molecules, metal-based compounds have unique physical, chemical and/ or biophysical properties. In this book chapter, we summarized the very recent progress (2013-2015) from the worldwide effort in the development of novel metal-based compounds. Some recent works on the anti-cancer studies of gold compounds including that of gold(I) and gold(III) will be discussed.

Keywords: Cancer, Cytotoxicity, Drugs, Encapsulation, Gold(I), Gold(III), *In vitro*, Medicine, Metal Complexes, MTT Assays.

INTRODUCTION

According to the recent released facts (February, 2015) from the World Health Organization (WHO), cancer is the leading cause of worldwide mortality, with approximately 8.2 million cancer-related deaths and 14 million new cases in year of 2012 [2]. It is also expected that the annual new cancer cases will rise to 22 the million within the next two decades. Although technological advancements

* **Corresponding author Raymond Wai-Yin Sun:** Flat D35 17/F, Block D, Wah Lok Industrial Centre Phase 2, 31-35 Shan Mei Street, Fotan, N. T., Hong Kong; Tel: (+852) 2319 9381; E-mail: rwysun@leemanchemical.com

Atta-ur-Rahman & M. Iqbal Choudhary (Eds.)

in surgery, cancer chemotherapeutics and radiotherapies have been achieved, cancer patients are not infrequently encountering problems associated with resistant cancer strains, cancer metastases and toxic/ harmful side effect from different types of anti-cancer treatments [3]. Moreover, the cancer facts tell us that there still remains a great urge in the discovery of new anti-cancer agents/ options for the treatment of cancers, especially for patients who are suffering from relapsed cancers. Inorganic compounds indeed open an avenue for new classes of anti-cancer agents since different metal compounds and their corresponding metal ions may have different sizes, charges, coordination geometries, ligand to metal binding kinetics, reactivity patterns in related to redox/ charge transfer, *etc.* [4]. Thus all these properties render metal compounds very often to have unique chemical, physical, biophysical and hence special (or favorable) biological and medical properties compared to conventional organic moieties [5].

In recent decades, a number of review articles have substantially covered the medicinal development of various metal-based drugs [5, 6]. This book chapter mainly focuses on the development of new metal-based drugs of gold in the recent three years (from 2013 to 2015).

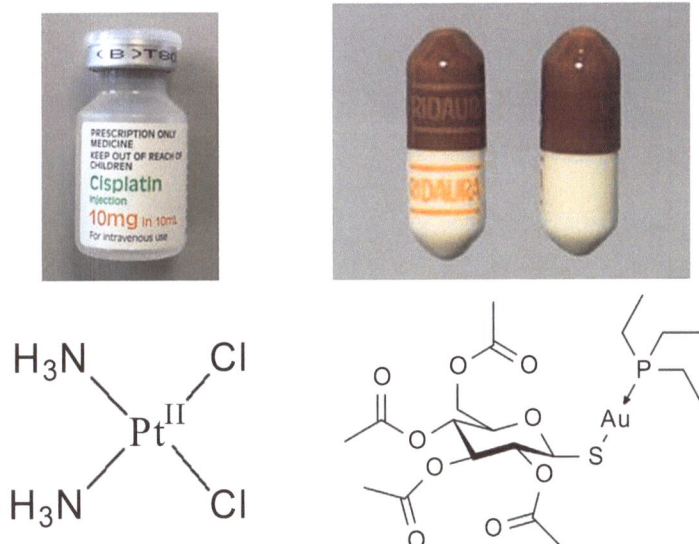

Fig. (1). Cisplatin (Left) and Auranofin (Right).

Gold Compounds

The oxidation states of gold exist from -1 to +5. In biological systems, the relative stable oxidation states include 0 [Au^0 or gold(0)], +1 [Au^I or gold(I)] and +3 [Au^{III} or gold(III)]. Gold compounds have a long history in medicinal chemistry for the treatment of tuberculosis and notably, rheumatoid arthritis. Since the discovery of the cytotoxic activities of a gold(I) compound (Auranofin, Fig. **1**) by Lorber and co-workers in 1979 [7], the anti-cancer properties of various gold(I) and gold(III) compounds have been uncovered afterwards [8]. Nevertheless, there are various factors hindering the medical development of gold compound to be used clinically. These factors include stability, solubility, toxicity, cancer-cell specificity and cellular uptake efficacy, *etc.* [9]. With the efforts contributed by researchers worldwide, various highly anti-cancer active gold(I) and gold(III) compounds have been identified [10]. Some of them even possess promising anti-tumor activities in animal studies.

Gold(I) Compounds

Since 1979, a number of gold(I) compounds have been identified to display anti-cancer activities [7]. Berners-Price and co-workers in the recent decade have developed a series of gold(I) carbene and phosphine compounds [11]. In 2013, she worked with Barnard *et al.* to discover a binuclear luminescent gold(I) N-heterocyclic carbene (NHC) compound which displays promising *in vitro* cytotoxicity [12]. By using fluorescence and X-ray absorption spectroscopy the anion binding capability of this compound were investigated (Fig. **2**).

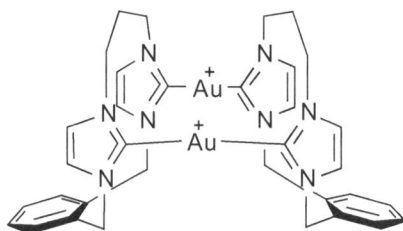

Fig. (2). Chemical structure of a gold(I) compound reported by Berners-Price, Barnard and co-workers [11].

Casini and co-workers in 2013 has re-investigated the anti-cancer property of Auranofin [13]. They found that this compound exerts inhibition effects of glutathione S-transferase P1-1 (GST P1-1) with a calculated IC_{50} value of 32.9 ± 0.5 I1/μM. According to the results from the inhibition assays of GST P1-1 and its cysteine mutants, the authors suggested that the cysteine residues are crucial for the enzyme inactivation in contrast to the reported inhibitors. Casini, Rigobello and co-workers have also developed various anti-cancer active gold(I) and silver(I) compounds containing ligands with a fluorescent anthracenyl ligand [14]. The gold compounds were found to induce oxidation of the thioredoxin system. With the fluorescent properties of the gold compounds, fluorescence microscopic study revealed that tumor cells have a much higher uptake rate of these compounds with respect to normal cells. Several caffeine-based gold(I) N-hetero-cyclic carbenes were identified as possible anticancer agents in 2014 (Fig. **3**) [15].

Among these compounds, a bis-carbene compound [Au(caffein-2- ylidene)$_2$][BF$_4$] was found to be highly selective for human ovarian cancer cell lines with no apparent toxicity to healthy organs at the effective dosages. This compound could act as an effective and selective G-quadruplex binder, and meanwhile, a modest PARP-1 inhibitor. A series of mono- and heterodinuclear gold(I) and platinum(II) compounds with a bipyridylamine-phosphine ligand have been reported by Casini, Bodio and co-workers in 2014 [16]. These compounds displayed a higher *in vitro* antiproliferative property and cellular uptake efficiency in cancer cells than cisplatin.

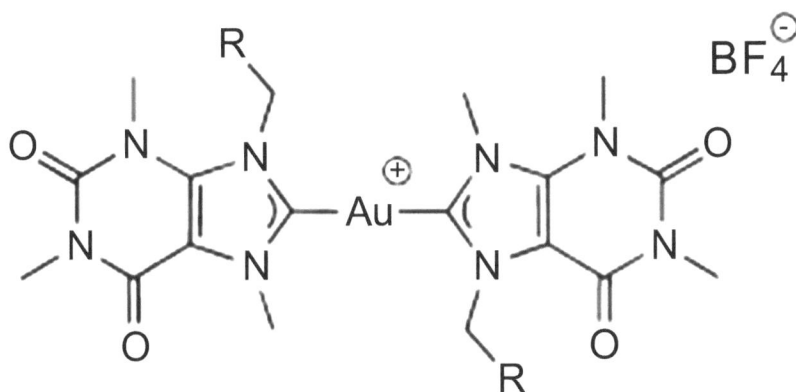

Fig. (3). Chemical structure of a kind of gold(I) compounds reported by Casini, Picquet and co-workers [15].

In addition to the heterodinuclear gold(I) and platinum(II) compounds, Casini, Bodio and co-workers in 2015 reported the anti-cancer activities of various homo- and heterobimetallic compounds of gold(I)-gold(I), gold(I)-copper(I) and gold(I)-ruthenium(II) [17]. These compounds were prepared *via* a novel microwave-assisted approach using gold(I) NHC compounds carrying a pentafluorophenol ester moiety. The *ex vivo* toxicity using the precision-cut tissue slices (PCTS) technique was examined. The inhibitory activities of these compounds towards seleno-enzyme thioredoxin reductase were found.

In 2014, Che and co-workers has identified a binuclear gold(I) compound with mixed bridging diphosphine and bis(N-heterocyclic carbene) ligands with potent *in vitro* and *in vivo* anti-cancer activities (Fig. **4**) [18]. This binuclear compound exhibits a favorable stability against serum albumin and could inhibit TrxR activity. *In vivo* studies showed that this compound could effectively inhibit tumor growth in mice bearing HeLa xenograft and mice bearing highly aggressive mouse B16-F10 melanoma. Moreover, it could inhibit angiogenesis in *in vivo* tumor models and sphere formation of cancer stem cells *in vitro*.

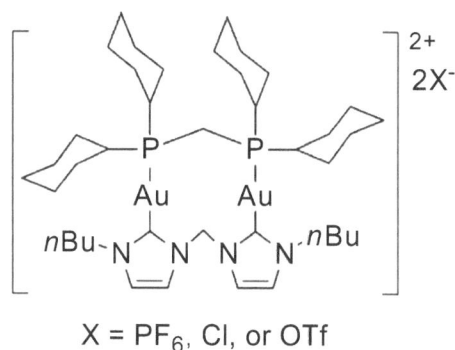

X = PF_6, Cl, or OTf

Fig. (4). Chemical structure of a binuclear gold(I) compound reported by Che and co-workers [18].

Gornitzka, Hemmer and co-workers in 2014 reported some new gold(I) compounds containing two 1-[2-(diethylamino)ethyl]imidazolydene ligands [19]. All these compounds showed *in vitro* antiproliferative activities toward prostate cancer cell line PC-3. Another new series of gold(I) compounds containing quinoline functionalized NHC(s) were also reported by the same research group in 2015 (Fig. **5**) [20]. These compounds as revealed from MTT assay displayed modest cytotoxic activities towards murine macrophages J774A.1. Nevertheless, this class of gold(I) compounds showed highly potent *in vitro* anti-leishmanial activity against *L. infantum promastigotes* and three of the gold(I) compounds also effectively inhibited *L. infantum* intracellular amastigotes.

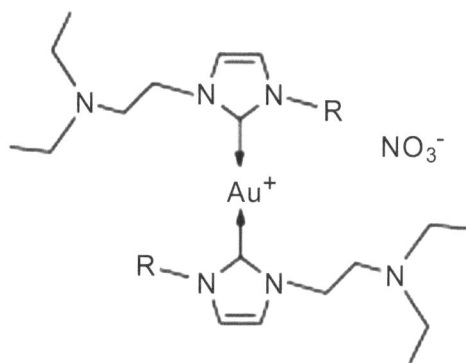

Fig. (5). Chemical structure of a gold(I) compound reported by Gornitzka, Hemmer and co-workers [20].

Mao and Liu in 2014 reported several gold(I) and silver(I) compounds containing NHCs derived from cyclophanes [21]. These compounds have a higher *in vitro* anti-cancer potency than the clinical-used cisplatin towards a cisplatin-resistant cell line. Intracellular distribution studies revealed that these compounds, particularly the gold(I) compounds, could selectively localize in the mitochondria of the cancer cells. The gold(I) compounds were found to induce both early apoptosis and late apoptosis *via* caspase- and ROS-dependent pathways.

Ott, Rodríguez and co-workers has reported some luminescent alkynyl-gold(I) coumarin derivatives and their anti-cancer activities in 2014 [22]. These compounds are water-soluble compounds containing water soluble phosphines. The presence of the gold(I) metal atom was suggested to be responsible for the increase of coumarin phosphorescence emission of these compounds. In general, the anionic analogs displayed stronger cytotoxic effects towards cancer cell lines than the neutral gold alkynyl compound. In contrast, significant inhibition with IC_{50} values of below 0.1 I1/μM of thioredoxin reductase (TrxR) was observed for the neutral compounds, while the anionic compounds were found to have IC_{50} values > 0.8 I1/μM. In the same year, Ott and co-workers have identified a series of gold(I) NHC compounds with phosphane ligands as potent inhibitors of various enzymes including seleno-enzyme thioredoxin reductase (TrxR) and of the zinc-finger enzyme poly(ADP-ribose) polymerase 1 (PARP-1) [23]. The inhibitory activities on TrxR were found to be depended on the length/ size of the alkyl/ aryl residues of phosphorus atoms. As revealed from density functional theory (DFT) calculations, the Au-P bond of the triphenylphosphane moieties $[Au^I(NHC)(PPh_3)]I$ had a lower bond dissociation energy compared to the trialkylphosphane moieties $[Au^I(NHC)(PR_3)]I$. These results indicated a higher kinetic reactivity of $[Au^I(NHC)(PPh_3)]I$.

Ott and co-workers in 2014 further developed various gold(I) NHC compounds with naphthalimide ligands as combined thioredoxin reductase inhibitors and DNA intercalators [24]. These organometallic conjugates were potent DNA intercalators owing to the presence of planar naphthalimide moieties. Meanwhile, the gold(I) moieties were believed to responsible for the Trx inhibition. More recently, Several gold(I) compounds with phosphane and thiotetrazolate ligands were found as highly efficient inhibitors of TrxR (Fig. **6**) [25]. These compounds displayed potent activities towards MDA-MB-231 breast adenocarcinoma, HT-29 colon carcinoma and notably, vincristine resistant Nalm-6 leukemia cells.

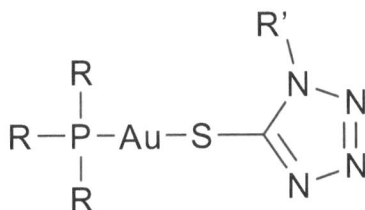

Fig. (6). Chemical structure of a gold(I) compound reported by Ott and co-workers [25].

In the collaboration with Wölfl, Ott and co-workers reported a detailed study of pro-apoptotic signaling and metabolic adaptation triggered by another gold(I)-NHC compound [triphenylphosphane-(1,3-diethyl-5-methoxy-benzylimid-zol-2-ylidene)] gold(I) iodide using quantitative signal transduction protein microarray analysis [26]. The results revealed that the induction of the strong cytotoxic effects and apoptosis of this compound were associated with an immediate and irreversible loss of mitochondrial respiration, and also by a crucial imbalance of the intracellular redox state. ELISA microarray analysis of signal transduction pathways suggested that thioredoxin reductase is one of the important targets for this gold(I) compound. The research team further reported that this TrxR inhibiting gold(I) compound could induce apoptosis through ASK1-p38-MAPK signaling in pancreatic cancer cells [27]. Biochemical assays revealed that this gold(I) compound is an effective TrxR inhibitor as well as an apoptosis inducer in gemcitabine-resistant pancreatic cancer cells *via* inhibition of Trx-ASK1-p38 signal cascade. In 2015, Ott collaborated with Serebryanskaya to develop a novel aminotriazole-based NHC compound [28]. This compound could trigger promising cytotoxic activities to breast cancer cells and effectively inhibit the activity of the enzyme thioredoxin reductase.

In order to gain a deeper insight into the molecular basis of TrxR inhibition and to prove the gold-selenocysteine coordination, Messori, Ott and co-workers have reported the investigation of some of the gold(I) NHC compounds with a synthetic C-terminal dodecapeptide of hTrxR containing Selenocysteine at position 498 by using electrospray ionization mass spectrometry (ESI-MS) [29]. Rapid formation of 1:1 Gold-peptide adducts in line with a quick inhibition of TrxR was found in all cases.

In 2015, Sun, Li and co-workers have developed a binuclear gold(I) pyrrolidinedithiocarbamato (PDTC) compound containing a bidentate carbene ligand (Fig. **7**) [30]. By MTT assay this compound shows promising cytotoxicity *in vitro* towards a cisplatin-resistant ovarian carcinoma cell line (A2780cis). Given that this gold(I) compound has high solution stability, its rigid scaffold enables a zinc(II)-based metal-organic framework (Zn-MOF) to be used as a carrier to facilitate its uptake and release under physiologically-relevant condition. Instead of using conventional dialysis approach for the drug-releasing testing, in this study we have designed and employed a set of TranswellA(r)-based experiments to examine the cytotoxic and antimigratory activities of 1@Zn-MOF towards the cisplatin-resistant ovarian cancer cells (A2780cis).

Tan, Leung and co-workers in 2015 have reported another series of diphosphine-dinuclear gold(I) compounds [31]. Two chiral gold(I) compounds containing methylester substituted diphosphine ligands were found to display significant anti-cancer activities and preference towards breast cancer cell lines MDA-M--231 and MCF10A. In the same year, Gimeno and co-workers have prepared a series of bioconjugated gold(I) compounds with cysteine-containing dipeptide [32]. Among these compounds, a compound with two $AuPPh_3^+$ moieties and a Boc-Cys-Gly-OMe peptide showed excellent cytotoxic activity towards a panel of cancer cell lines with IC_{50} values in the very low micromolar range (as low as 0.1 μM).

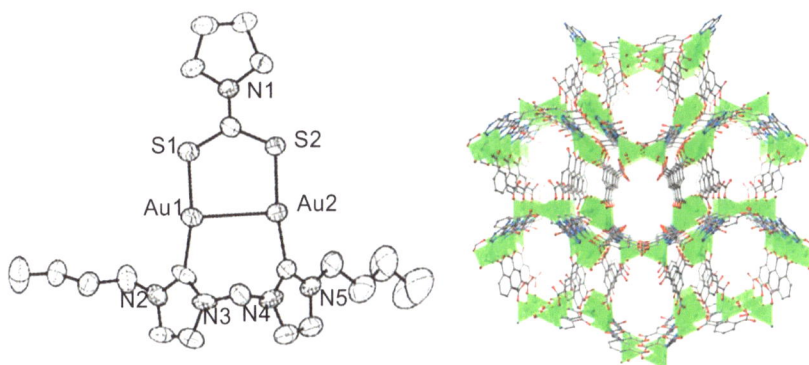

Fig. (7). The crystal structure of a binuclear gold(I) dithiocarbamate complex (Left) and a zinc-based metal-organic framework (Zn-MOF, Right) reported by Sun, Li and co-workers [30].

Gold(III) Compounds

Being iso-structural to platinum(II) compounds, gold(III) compounds have long been regarded as effective analogues of cisplatin. However, under physiological condition, gold(III) ion is easily to be reduced to gold(I) or gold(0). Thus one of the major challenges for the development of gold(III) medicines is this stability issue. In the recent decade, various gold(III) compounds with potent anti-cancer properties have been identified and developed by using various kinds of bidentate, tridentate or tetradentate ligands.

Casini and co-workers in 2013 have reported the use of some anti-cancer gold(III) compounds to achieve inhibition of membrane water/ glycerol channels of aquaporin protein [33]. Various gold(III) compounds bearing nitrogen donor ligands including 1,10-phenatroline, 2,2'-bipyridine, 4,4'-dimethyl-2,2'-bipyridine, 4,4'-diamino-2,2'-bipyridine and 2,2';6',2"-terpyridine have been evaluated in human red blood cells expressing AQP1 and AQP3, which are responsible for water and glycerol movement, respectively. By means of a stopped-flow method, the gold(III) compounds were found to selectively modulate AQP3 over AQP1. At the same year, Contel, Casini and co-workers have identified various heterometallic gold(III)-iron compounds with iminophosphorane ligands showing anti-cancer activities (Fig. **8**) [34]. These compounds have antiproliferative activities towards human ovarian cancer cells A2780 and its cisplatin-resistant strain (A2780S/R). Notably, among these compounds, the trimetallic derivative Au$_2$Fe showed higher cytotoxicity than its monometallic fragments. Moreover, studies of the interactions of this trimetallic compound with DNA and the zinc-finger protein PARP-1 revealed that this compound could exert different mechanisms of actions with respect to cisplatin.

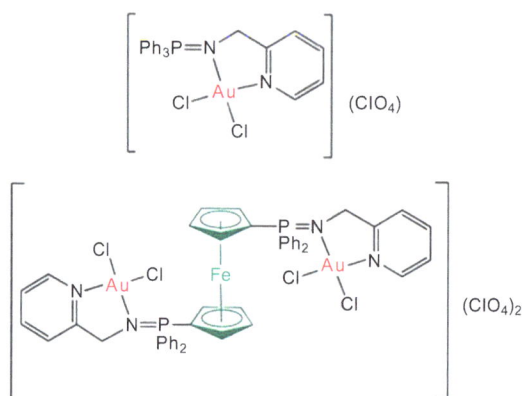

Fig. (8). Chemical structures of a gold(III) mononuclear compound and a heterometallic gold(III)-iron compound prepared by Casini, Contel and co-workers [34].

In 2003, Che and co-workers have first reported the anti-cancer properties of a series of physiologically stable gold(III) porphyrin compounds [35]. Some of these compounds including the gold(III) *meso*-tetraphenylporphyrin compound (gold-**1a**, Fig. **9**) have subsequently been found to possess promising *in vitro* and *in vivo* anti-cancer activities in the recent 12 years. In 2013, Che and Sun have first reported that the gold(III) compound is capable to display anti-cancer properties towards cancer stem cells [36]. The gold-**1a** was found to block the self-renewal ability of cancer stem-like cells and show appealing safety pharmacological profiles in rodents. In 2014, the gold-**1a** has been reported to effectively inhibit the growth of cisplatin-resistant ovarian cancer cells (A2780cis) in association with upregulation of a proapoptotic gene *PMS2*, which has a DNA mismatch repair and proapoptotic functions [37]. At the same year, Che has designed a cancer-targeted nanosystem for delivery of the gold(III) porphyrin compound with enhanced selectivity and apoptosis-inducing efficacy [38]. Cancer-targeted mesoporous silica nanoparticles (MSN) were designed to delivery gold-**1a** to cancer cells and amplify the inhibitory effects towards thioredoxin reductase (TrxR) of gold-**1a**.

In 2010, Che and co-workers also developed 25 novel gold(III) porphyrin compounds including some water-soluble and asymmetrical compounds with a dynamic range of lipophilicity [39]. In general the higher the lipophilicity of the compounds, the higher the cytotoxic activities were observed. Sessler and co-workers in 2015 have identified a series of new water-soluble gold(III) porphyrin compounds with cytotoxic IC_{50} values down to 9 μM [40].

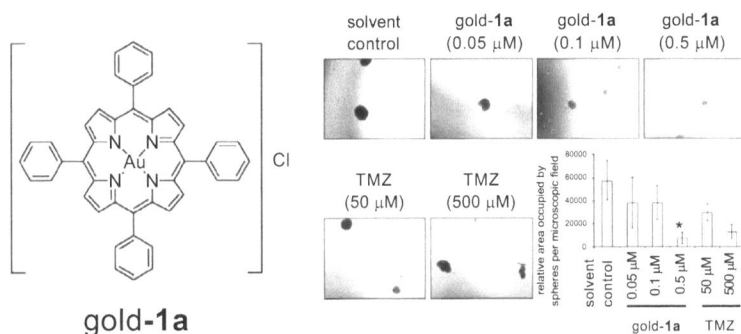

Fig. (9). Chemical structure of a gold(III) tetraphenylporphyrinato compound (gold-**1a**) and its anti-cancer stem cells activities revealed by the sphere formation assay [36].

Apart from gold(III) porphyrin compounds, Che and co-workers have also developed other classes of anti-cancer active gold(III) compounds. This research team has developed various gold(III) compounds containing N-heterocyclic carbene ligands to be used as effective thiol "switch-on" fluorescent probes [41]. Some of these compounds have also displayed promising *in vitro* and *in vivo* anti-cancer properties. Another new class of gold(III) carbene compounds containing various bidentate C-deprotonated C^N and cis-chelating bis(N-heterocyclic carbene) (bis-NHC) ligands has been synthesized and characterized [42]. These compounds have good solubility in water and are the first examples of gold(III) compounds supported by bis-NHC ligands to display emission in solutions under degassed condition at room temperature with emission maxima (λ_{max}) at 498-633 nm and emission quantum yields of up to 10.1%. One of these water-soluble gold(III) compounds was found to display a significant inhibitory activity towards deubiquitinase (DUB) UCHL3 with IC_{50} value of 0.15 μM.

Another classes of gold(III) compound with dithiocarbamate ligands $[Au^{III}(C^\wedge N)(R_2NCS_2)]^+$ (whereas HC^N = 2-phenylpyridine) have also been developed by the same group [43]. These compounds were found to display significant inhibition on deubiquitinases (DUBs), and showed high selective *in vitro* cytotoxicity towards breast cancer cells which are correlated to the high cellular uptake of gold as demonstrated by ICP-MS study. These compounds were also found to induce cell-cycle arrest, apoptosis, and have anti-angiogenic pro-perty that could be related to the DUB inhibitory activities. Che and co-workers in

2013 also developed various gold(III) allenylidene compounds with phosphorescence properties [44]. These compounds are readily self-assembled to form nanostructures in solution and display cytotoxicity towards cancer cells.

A physiologically stable gold(III) phosphine compound [(C^N^C)$_2$Au$_2$(μ-dppp)](CF$_3$SO$_3$)$_2$ [**Au3**, HC^N^CH= 2,6-diphenylpyridine; dppp= bis(diphenyl-phosphino)propane] have been identified in 2013 by Che and co-workers and was found to display prominent *in vitro* cytotoxicity towards various cancers having sub-micromolar range cytotoxic IC$_{50}$ values (Fig. **10**) [45]. This compound was shown to have promising inhibition on tumor growth *in vivo*, and exert low acute and sub-chronic toxicities in mice and beagle dogs. Transcriptomic and connectivity map analyses suggested that the transcriptional profile of this compound is similar to those thioredoxin reductase (TrxR) inhibitor and endoplasmic reticulum (ER) stress inducers. The transcriptomic analysis also revealed **Au3** could induce expression of death receptor 5 (DR5) in cancer cells. Since recombinant protein TRAIL could interact with DR5 and induce apoptosis in cancer cells, thus TRAIL could be used and hence, has been proven to be an effective synergistic agent to improve the anti-tumor activity of **Au3**. Very recently, the same research group have developed a luminescent cyclometalated gold(III)-avidin conjugate having a long-lived emissive excited state of 1.8 µs in PBS solution in open air [46]. This compound could be used as luminescent dye to stain various proteins and DNA.

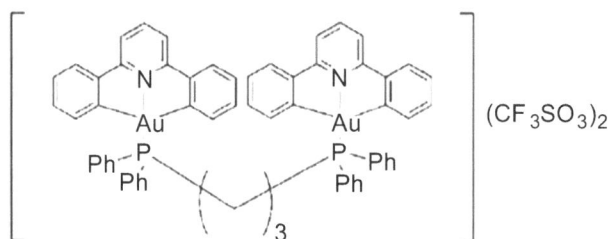

Fig. (10). Chemical structure of a physiologically stable gold(III) phosphine compound [(C^N^C)$_2$Au$_2$($A\mu$-dppp)](CF$_3$SO$_3$)$_2$ [**Au3**, HC^N^CH= 2,6-diphenylpyridine; dppp= bis(diphenylphosphino)propane reported by Che and Sun [45].

Since the discovery of the anti-cancer properties of a gold(III) dithiocarbamate compound in 2005, various gold(III) dithiocarbamato derivatives have been developed in the recent ten years [47]. Some of these dithiocarbamate compounds contain amino acids or oligopeptides have been reported to display promising anti-cancer properties. Yet, most of the capability in interacting with biologically relevant molecules remains poorly understood. In 2013, Fregona and co-workers have examined the affinity of several gold(III) dithiocarbamate compounds with chemical formula of [Au^{III}Br$_2$(dtc-Sar-OCH$_3$)] (whereas dtc: dithiocarbamate; Sar:

sarcosine (N-methylglycine)) with some biomolecules such as histidine-, methionine-, and cysteine-rich proteins, *etc.* [48].

In the collaboration with Dou, Fregona and co-workers have developed several gold(III) dithiocarbamato peptidomimetics as promising anti-cancer agents against human breast neoplasia (Fig. **11**) [49]. These compounds show improved chemotherapeutic index and therapeutic spectrum. Some of these compounds are highly active towards human MDA-MB-231 (resistant to cisplatin) breast cancer cell cultures and xenografts. Proteasomes were identified to be the potential target of these novel gold(III) compounds. Very recently, Fregona and co-workers have developed various gold(III) pyrrolidinedithiocarbamato (PDTC) compounds, namely [Au^{III}Br$_2$(PDTC)] and [Au^{III}Cl$_2$(PDTC)] as promising anti-cancer agents [50]. They found that the bromide derivative was more effective than the chloride one in terms of IC$_{50}$ values to the cancer cells and the capability in inducing apoptotic cell death for a series of cancer cell lines. The bromide derivative would induce oxidative stress and exert effects on the permeability transition pore, a mitochondrial channel whose opening leads to cell death.

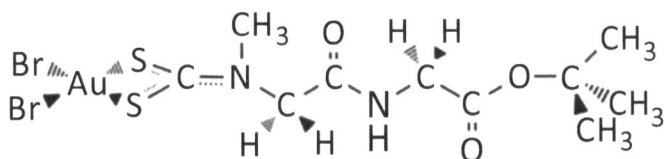

Fig. (11). Chemical structure of a typical gold(III) dithiocarbamate peptidomimetic prepared by Fregona, Dou and co-workers [49].

To improve the stability and cancer cell selectivity of the gold(III) dithiocarbamato compounds, Accardo and Fregona *et al.* have prepared target selective micelles for bombesin receptors to encapsulate the gold(III) compounds [51]. They developed some sterically stabilized micelles (SSM) of DSPE-PEG2000, as well as sterically stabilized mixed micelles (SSMM) having PC or DOPC phospholipids (5, 10 or 20% mol/mol with respect to DSPE-PEG2000) as delivery systems for the gold(III) dithiocarbamate compounds, By means of UV-vis spectrophotometry, the gold(III) compounds were found to be stable under physiologically relevant conditions for 72 h. Incorporation in micelle composition of a low amount of the peptide derivative MonY-BN-AA1, containing a bombesin peptide analogue does not change the size of the micelles. Targeting selective properties of these micelles were confirmed by using PC-3 cells over expressing the GRP/ bombesin receptors.

Since 2006, Messori and co-workers have developed a series of binuclear gold(III)-oxo compounds and have examined their anti-cancer activities *in vitro*

[52]. One of these compounds (namely oxo-6, Fig. **12**) was found to be highly anti-cancer active towards a panel of cancer cell lines and display a high cancer-cell selectivity. In 2014, the interaction between this promising gold(III) compound and some biologically relevant molecules have been examined by this research team [53]. By means of X-ray diffraction and ESI mass spectrometry, the gold adducts of the protein bovine pancreatic ribonuclease and thioredoxin reductase have been characterized. In addition to the oxo-6, another anti-cancer active binuclear gold(III)-oxo compound (namely Auoxo3) has been examined for the interaction with the protein lysozyme [54]. By means of X-ray crystallography, UV-Vis absorption spectroscopy and circular dichroism (CD), the Auoxo3 were found to be disintegrated. The gold(III) metal center would undergo reduction and produce reactive gold(I) species which are capable to bind with the protein and hence form a relative stable derivatives.

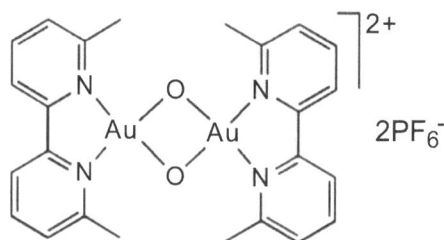

Fig. (12). Chemical structure of a binuclear oxo-bridged gold(III) compound (**Auoxo-6**) prepared by Messori and co-workers [52].

In 2000, an organogold(III) compound Aubipy[c] has been identified to display highly potent anti-proliferative properties *in vitro* [55]. In 2014, a classical proteomic approach including the use of 2-D gel electrophoresis separation and subsequent mass spectrometry identification has been launched by Messori and co-workers in order to elucidate the action mechanisms of this gold(III) compound in A2780 human ovarian cancer cells [56]. Bioinformatic analysis of the altered proteins revealed that this gold(III) compound primarily perturbs mitochondrial processes and the glycolytic pathway in the cancer cells. These data suggested a new action mechanism of the gold(III) drug. The same research group in 2014 has also successfully obtained the crystal structure by X-ray crystallography of the complex formed when a protein hen egg white enzyme lysozyme reacts with Aubipy[c] [57]. As revealed from the crystal structure, it is believed that the gold(III) compound after interacting with HEWL, undergoes reduction of the gold(III) center followed by detaching of the cyclometalated ligand.

In 2014, Vasic, Messori and co-workers have examined the effect of various gold(III) compounds on Na(+)/ K(+)-ATPase [58]. This enzyme is responsible for maintaining the intracellular ionic and osmotic balance by using ATP as an energy source to pump excess sodium ions out of the cell in exchange for potassium ions. Three representative cytotoxic gold(III) compounds including [Au(bipy) (OH)$_2$][PF$_6$] (whereas bipy = 2,2'-bipyridine), [Au(py(dmb)-H) (CH$_3$COO)$_2$] (whereas py(dmb)-H = deprotonated 6-(1,1-dimethylbenzyl)-pyridine), and [Au(bipy(dmb)-H)(OH)][PF$_6$] (whereas bipy(dmb)-H = deprotonated 6-(1,1-dimethylbenzyl)-2,2'-bipyridine) were found to interfere with this enzyme. The examined gold(III) compounds were found to display a pronounced, non-competitive and reversible inhibition on Na(+)/ (+)-ATPase. Notably, the authors showed that treatment with cysteine (Cys) resulted in the prevention of enzyme.

In addition to the anti-cancer properties, Messori and co-workers in 2013 also identified several gold(III) and gold(I) compounds displaying anti-lesishmanial activities [59]. Trypanothione reductase (TR) is a possible drug target for antileishmanial agents and based on the efforts from this research team, a group of structurally diverse gold compounds were also found to have promising inhibition on TR *in vitro*.

CONCLUDING REMARKS

The rich coordination chemistry of metal ions render metal compounds including that of gold(I) and gold(III) to have diverse structures and unique chemical and biological properties. From 2013 to 2015, several classes of novel gold(I) and gold(III) compounds have already been developed and most of them, showed promising *in vitro* and even *in vivo* anti-cancer properties. Based on the recent studies, the underlying modes of action of some gold(I) and gold(III) compounds were believed to be the inhibition of the enzyme thioredoxin reductase TrxR or other thiol-containing proteins. Great efforts have already been made by numerous scientists working towards novel gold medicines. Together with the gold(III) compounds showing promising *in vitro*, *in vivo* anti-cancer properties and also the unique mode of action to the cancer cells, we anticipate that in the coming ten years some gold compounds will be entered clinical trials especially for the treatment of drug-resistant and relapsed cancers.

CONFLICT OF INTEREST

The authors declares no conflict of interest, financial or otherwise.

ACKNOWLEDGEMENTS

This work was supported by Shantou University Start-Up Fund, (2013 NTF13005) and the General Research Fund (HKU 704812P) administrated by

University Grants Council (HKSAR, China). The authors thank the technical support from Ms. Jun-Jiao Zhou.

REFERENCES

[1]   a) Rosenberg B, Vancamp L, Krigas T. Inhibition of cell division in Escherichia coli by electrolysis products from a platinum electrode. Nature 1965; 205: 698-9.
[http://dx.doi.org/10.1038/205698a0] [PMID: 14287410] ; b) Rosenberg B, VanCamp L, Trosko JE, Mansour VH. Platinum compounds: a new class of potent antitumour agents. Nature 1969; 222(5191): 385-6.
[http://dx.doi.org/10.1038/222385a0] [PMID: 5782119]

[2]   Recent statistic on cancers from the World Health Organization (http://www.who.int/-mediacentre/factsheets/fs297/en/).

[3]   Holohan C, Van Schaeybroeck S, Longley DB, Johnston PG. Cancer drug resistance: an evolving paradigm. Nat Rev Cancer 2013; 13(10): 714-26.
[http://dx.doi.org/10.1038/nrc3599] [PMID: 24060863]

[4]   Thompson KH, Orvig C. Boon and bane of metal ions in medicine. Science 2003; 300(5621): 936-9.
[http://dx.doi.org/10.1126/science.1083004] [PMID: 12738851]

[5]   a) Che CM, Siu FM. Metal complexes in medicine with a focus on enzyme inhibition. Curr Opin Chem Biol 2010; 14(2): 255-61.
[http://dx.doi.org/10.1016/j.cbpa.2009.11.015] [PMID: 20018553] ; b) Barry NP, Sadler PJ. Challenges for metals in medicine: how nanotechnology may help to shape the future. ACS Nano 2013; 7(7): 5654-9.
[http://dx.doi.org/10.1021/nn403220e] [PMID: 23837396] ; c) Medici S, Peana M, Nurchi VM, Lachowicz JI, Crisponi G, Zoroddu MA. Noble metals in medicine: Latest advances. Coord Chem Rev 2015; 284: 329-50.
[http://dx.doi.org/10.1016/j.ccr.2014.08.002]

[6]   a) Ott I, Gust R. Non platinum metal complexes as anti-cancer drugs. Arch Pharm (Weinheim) 2007; 340(3): 117-26.
[http://dx.doi.org/10.1002/ardp.200600151] [PMID: 17315259] ; b) Sun RW, Ma DL, Wong EL, Che CM. Some uses of transition metal complexes as anti-cancer and anti-HIV agents. Dalton Trans 2007; (43): 4884-92.
[PMID: 17992273] ; c) Desoize B. Metals and metal compounds in cancer treatment. Anticancer Res 2004; 24(3a): 1529-44.
[PMID: 15274320]

[7]   Simon TM, Kunishima DH, Vibert GJ, Lorber A. Inhibitory effects of a new oral gold compound on HeLa cells. Cancer 1979; 44(6): 1965.
[http://dx.doi.org/10.1002/1097-0142(197912)44:6<1965::AID-CNCR2820440602>3.0.CO;2-6] [PMID: 389401]

[8]   Shaw CF III. Gold-based therapeutic agents. Chem Rev 1999; 99(9): 2589-600.
[http://dx.doi.org/10.1021/cr980431o] [PMID: 11749494]

[9]   Sun RW. Strategies to improve the anti-cancer properties of gold(III) complexes. Modern Chem Appl 2013; 1: 102.
[http://dx.doi.org/10.4172/mca.1000102]

[10]   a) Che CM, Sun RW. Therapeutic applications of gold complexes: lipophilic gold(III) cations and gold(I) complexes for anti-cancer treatment. Chem Commun (Camb) 2011; 47(34): 9554-60.
[http://dx.doi.org/10.1039/c1cc10860c] [PMID: 21674082] ; b) Ott I. On the medicinal chemistry of gold complexes as anticancer drugs. Coord Chem Rev 2009; 253: 1670-81.
[http://dx.doi.org/10.1016/j.ccr.2009.02.019]

[11]   Berners-Price SJ, Filipovska A. Gold compounds as therapeutic agents for human diseases.

Metallomics 2011; 3(9): 863-73.
[http://dx.doi.org/10.1039/c1mt00062d] [PMID: 21755088]

[12] Wedlock LE, Aitken JB, Berners-Price SJ, Barnard PJ. Bromide ion binding by a dinuclear gold(I) N-heterocyclic carbene complex: a spectrofluorescence and X-ray absorption spectroscopic study. Dalton Trans 2013; 42(4): 1259-66.
[http://dx.doi.org/10.1039/C2DT31817B] [PMID: 23138339]

[13] De Luca A, Hartinger CG, Dyson PJ, Lo Bello M, Casini A. A new target for gold(I) compounds: glutathione-S-transferase inhibition by auranofin. J Inorg Biochem 2013; 119: 38-42.
[http://dx.doi.org/10.1016/j.jinorgbio.2012.08.006] [PMID: 23183361]

[14] Citta A, Schuh E, Mohr F, *et al.* Fluorescent silver(I) and gold(I)-N-heterocyclic carbene complexes with cytotoxic properties: mechanistic insights. Metallomics 2013; 5(8): 1006-15.
[http://dx.doi.org/10.1039/c3mt20260g] [PMID: 23661165]

[15] Bertrand B, Stefan L, Pirrotta M, *et al.* Caffeine-based gold(I) N-heterocyclic carbenes as possible anticancer agents: synthesis and biological properties. Inorg Chem 2014; 53(4): 2296-303.
[http://dx.doi.org/10.1021/ic403011h] [PMID: 24499428]

[16] Wenzel M, Bigaeva E, Richard P, *et al.* New heteronuclear gold(I)-platinum(II) complexes with cytotoxic properties: are two metals better than one? J Inorg Biochem 2014; 141: 10-6.
[http://dx.doi.org/10.1016/j.jinorgbio.2014.07.011] [PMID: 25172993]

[17] Bertrand B, Citta A, Franken IL, *et al.* Gold(I) NHC-based homo- and heterobimetallic complexes: synthesis, characterization and evaluation as potential anticancer agents. J Biol Inorg Chem 2015; 20(6): 1005-20.
[http://dx.doi.org/10.1007/s00775-015-1283-1] [PMID: 26202908]

[18] Zou T, Lum CT, Lok CN, To WP, Low KH, Che CM. A binuclear gold(I) complex with mixed bridging diphosphine and bis(N-heterocyclic carbene) ligands shows favorable thiol reactivity and inhibits tumor growth and angiogenesis *in vivo*. Angew Chem Int Ed Engl 2014; 53(23): 5810-4.
[http://dx.doi.org/10.1002/anie.201400142] [PMID: 24729298]

[19] Boselli L, Ader I, Carraz M, Hemmert C, Cuvillier O, Gornitzka H. Synthesis, structures, and selective toxicity to cancer cells of gold(I) complexes involving N-heterocyclic carbene ligands. Eur J Med Chem 2014; 85: 87-94.
[http://dx.doi.org/10.1016/j.ejmech.2014.07.086] [PMID: 25078312]

[20] Paloque L, Hemmert C, Valentin A, Gornitzka H. Synthesis, characterization, and antileishmanial activities of gold(I) complexes involving quinoline functionalized N-heterocyclic carbenes. Eur J Med Chem 2015; 94: 22-9.
[http://dx.doi.org/10.1016/j.ejmech.2015.02.046] [PMID: 25747497]

[21] Li Y, Liu GF, Tan CP, Ji LN, Mao ZW. Antitumor properties and mechanisms of mitochondria-targeted Ag(I) and Au(I) complexes containing N-heterocyclic carbenes derived from cyclophanes. Metallomics 2014; 6(8): 1460-8.
[http://dx.doi.org/10.1039/C4MT00046C] [PMID: 24788133]

[22] Arcau J, Andermark V, Aguil A3 E, *et al.* Luminescent alkynyl-gold(I) coumarin derivatives and their biological activity. Dalton Trans 2014; 43(11): 4426-36.
[http://dx.doi.org/10.1039/C3DT52594E] [PMID: 24302256]

[23] Rubbiani R, Salassa L, de Almeida A, Casini A, Ott I. Cytotoxic gold(I) N-heterocyclic carbene complexes with phosphane ligands as potent enzyme inhibitors. ChemMedChem 2014; 9(6): 1205-10.
[http://dx.doi.org/10.1002/cmdc.201400056] [PMID: 24677779]

[24] Meyer A, Oehninger L, Geldmacher Y, *et al.* Gold(I) N-heterocyclic carbene complexes with naphthalimide ligands as combined thioredoxin reductase inhibitors and DNA intercalators. ChemMedChem 2014; 9(8): 1794-800.
[PMID: 24803348]

[25]   Serebryanskaya TV, Lyakhov AS, Ivashkevich LS, *et al.* Gold(I) thiotetrazolates as thioredoxin reductase inhibitors and antiproliferative agents. Dalton Trans 2015; 44(3): 1161-9.
[http://dx.doi.org/10.1039/C4DT03105A] [PMID: 25413270]

[26]   Holenya P, Can S, Rubbiani R, *et al.* Detailed analysis of pro-apoptotic signaling and metabolic adaptation triggered by a N-heterocyclic carbene-gold(I) complex. Metallomics 2014; 6(9): 1591-601.
[http://dx.doi.org/10.1039/C4MT00075G] [PMID: 24777153]

[27]   Cheng X, Holenya P, Can S, *et al.* A TrxR inhibiting gold(I) NHC complex induces apoptosis through ASK1-p38-MAPK signaling in pancreatic cancer cells. Mol Cancer 2014; 13: 221.
[http://dx.doi.org/10.1186/1476-4598-13-221] [PMID: 25253202]

[28]   Serebryanskaya TV, Zolotarev AA, Ott I. A novel aminotriazole-based NHC complex for the design of gold(I) anti-cancer agents: synthesis and biological evaluation. MedChemComm 2015; 6: 1186-9.
[http://dx.doi.org/10.1039/C5MD00185D]

[29]   Pratesi A, Gabbiani C, Michelucci E, *et al.* Insights on the mechanism of thioredoxin reductase inhibition by gold N-heterocyclic carbene compounds using the synthetic linear selenocysteine containing C-terminal peptide hTrxR(488499): an ESI-MS investigation. J Inorg Biochem 2014; 136: 161-9.
[http://dx.doi.org/10.1016/j.jinorgbio.2014.01.009] [PMID: 24524917]

[30]   Sun RW, Zhang M, Li D, *et al.* Dinuclear gold(I) pyrrolidinedithiocarbamato complex: Cytotoxic and antimigratory activities on cancer cells and the use of metal-organic framework. Chemistry 2015; 21(51): 18534-8.
[http://dx.doi.org/10.1002/chem.201503656] [PMID: 26459298]

[31]   Li BB, Jia YX, Zhu PC, *et al.* Highly selective anti-cancer properties of ester functionalized enantiopure dinuclear gold(I)-diphosphine. Eur J Med Chem 2015; 98: 250-5.
[http://dx.doi.org/10.1016/j.ejmech.2015.05.027] [PMID: 26047407]

[32]   GutiA(c)rrez A, Marzo I, Cativiela C, Laguna A, Gimeno MC. Highly cytotoxic bioconjugated gold(I) complexes with cysteine-containing dipeptides. Chemistry 2015; 21(31): 11088-95.
[http://dx.doi.org/10.1002/chem.201501458] [PMID: 26111275]

[33]   Martins AP, Ciancetta A, de Almeida A, *et al.* Aquaporin inhibition by gold(III) compounds: new insights. ChemMedChem 2013; 8(7): 1086-92.
[http://dx.doi.org/10.1002/cmdc.201300107] [PMID: 23653381]

[34]   Lease N, Vasilevski V, Carreira M, *et al.* Potential anticancer heterometallic Fe-Au and Fe-Pd agents: initial mechanistic insights. J Med Chem 2013; 56(14): 5806-18.
[http://dx.doi.org/10.1021/jm4007615] [PMID: 23786413]

[35]   Che CM, Sun RW, Yu WY, Ko CB, Zhu N, Sun H. Gold(III) porphyrins as a new class of anticancer drugs: cytotoxicity, DNA binding and induction of apoptosis in human cervix epitheloid cancer cells. Chem Commun (Camb) 2003; (14): 1718-9.
[http://dx.doi.org/10.1039/b303294a] [PMID: 12877519]

[36]   Lum CT, Wong AS, Lin MC, Che CM, Sun RW. A gold(III) porphyrin complex as an anti-cancer candidate to inhibit growth of cancer-stem cells. Chem Commun (Camb) 2013; 49(39): 4364-6.
[http://dx.doi.org/10.1039/C2CC37366A] [PMID: 23223325]

[37]   Lum CT, Sun RW, Zou T, Che CM. Gold(III) complexes inhibit growth of cisplatin-resistant ovarian cancer in association with upregulation of proapoptotic PMS2 gene. Chem Sci (Camb) 2014; 5(4): 1579-84.
[http://dx.doi.org/10.1039/c3sc53203h]

[38]   He L, Chen T, You Y, *et al.* A cancer-targeted nanosystem for delivery of gold(III) complexes: enhanced selectivity and apoptosis-inducing efficacy of a gold(III) porphyrin complex. Angew Chem Int Ed Engl 2014; 53(46): 12532-6.
[PMID: 25220408]

[39] Sun RW, Li CK, Ma DL, *et al.* Stable anticancer gold(III)-porphyrin complexes: effects of porphyrin structure. Chemistry 2010; 16(10): 3097-113.
[http://dx.doi.org/10.1002/chem.200902741] [PMID: 20162647]

[40] Lammer AD, Cook ME, Sessler JL. Synthesis and anti-cancer activities of a water soluble gold(III) porphyrin. J Porphyr Phthalocyanines 2015; 19(1-03): 398-403.
[http://dx.doi.org/10.1142/S1088424615500236] [PMID: 25914517]

[41] Zou T, Lum CT, Chui SS, Che CM. Gold(III) complexes containing N-heterocyclic carbene ligands: thiol switch-on fluorescent probes and anti-cancer agents. Angew Chem Int Ed Engl 2013; 52(10): 2930-3.
[http://dx.doi.org/10.1002/anie.201209787] [PMID: 23371740]

[42] Hung FF, To WP, Zhang JJ, Ma C, Wong WY, Che CM. Water-soluble luminescent cyclometalated gold(III) complexes with cis-chelating bis(N-heterocyclic carbene) ligands: synthesis and photophysical properties. Chemistry 2014; 20(28): 8604-14.
[http://dx.doi.org/10.1002/chem.201403103] [PMID: 24957269]

[43] Zhang JJ, Ng KM, Lok CN, Sun RW, Che CM. Deubiquitinases as potential anti-cancer targets for gold(III) complexes. Chem Commun (Camb) 2013; 49(45): 5153-5.
[http://dx.doi.org/10.1039/c3cc41766b] [PMID: 23629480]

[44] Xiao XS, Kwong WL, Guan X, Yang C, Lu W, Che CM. Platinum(II) and gold(III) allenylidene complexes: phosphorescence, self-assembled nanostructures and cytotoxicity. Chemistry 2013; 19(29): 9457-62.
[http://dx.doi.org/10.1002/chem.201301481] [PMID: 23780563]

[45] Sun RW, Lok CN, Fong TT, *et al.* A dinuclear cyclometalated gold(III)-phosphine complex targeting thioredoxin reductase inhibits hepatocellular carcinoma *in vivo*. Chem Sci (Camb) 2013; 4(5): 1979-88.
[http://dx.doi.org/10.1039/c3sc21972k]

[46] Tsai JL, Chan AO, Che CM. A luminescent cyclometalated gold(iii)-avidin conjugate with a long-lived emissive excited state that binds to proteins and DNA and possesses anti-proliferation capacity. Chem Commun (Camb) 2015; 51(40): 8547-50.
[http://dx.doi.org/10.1039/C5CC00186B] [PMID: 25896112]

[47] Ronconi L, Aldinucci D, Dou QP, Fregona D. Latest insights into the anticancer activity of gold(III)-dithiocarbamato complexes. Anticancer Agents Med Chem 2010; 10(4): 283-92.
[http://dx.doi.org/10.2174/187152010791162298] [PMID: 20184554]

[48] Boscutti G, MarchiA□ L, Ronconi L, Fregona D. Insights into the reactivity of gold-dithiocarbamato anticancer agents toward model biomolecules by using multinuclear NMR spectroscopy. Chemistry 2013; 19(40): 13428-36.
[http://dx.doi.org/10.1002/chem.201302550] [PMID: 24038383]

[49] Nardon C, Schmitt SM, Yang H, Zuo J, Fregona D, Dou QP. Gold(III)-dithiocarbamato peptidomimetics in the forefront of the targeted anticancer therapy: preclinical studies against human breast neoplasia. PLoS One 2014; 9(1): e84248.
[http://dx.doi.org/10.1371/journal.pone.0084248] [PMID: 24392119]

[50] Nardon C, Chiara F, Brustolin L, *et al.* Gold(III)-pyrrolidinedithiocarbamato derivatives as antineoplastic agents. ChemistryOpen 2015; 4(2): 183-91.
[http://dx.doi.org/10.1002/open.201402091] [PMID: 25969817]

[51] Ringhieri P, Iannitti R, Nardon C, *et al.* Target selective micelles for bombesin receptors incorporating Au(III)-dithiocarbamato complexes. Int J Pharm 2014; 473(1-2): 194-202.
[http://dx.doi.org/10.1016/j.ijpharm.2014.07.014] [PMID: 25014371]

[52] Nobili S, Mini E, Landini I, Gabbiani C, Casini A, Messori L. Gold compounds as anticancer agents: chemistry, cellular pharmacology, and preclinical studies. Med Res Rev 2010; 30(3): 550-80.

[PMID: 19634148]

[53] Messori L, Scaletti F, Massai L, *et al.* Interactions of gold-based drugs with proteins: crystal structure of the adduct formed between ribonuclease A and a cytotoxic gold(III) compound. Metallomics 2014; 6(2): 233-6.
[http://dx.doi.org/10.1039/C3MT00265A] [PMID: 24287583]

[54] Russo Krauss I, Messori L, Cinellu MA, Marasco D, Sirignano R, Merlino A. Interactions of gold-based drugs with proteins: the structure and stability of the adduct formed in the reaction between lysozyme and the cytotoxic gold(III) compound Auoxo3. Dalton Trans 2014; 43(46): 17483-8.
[http://dx.doi.org/10.1039/C4DT02332C] [PMID: 25340580]

[55] Messori L, Abbate F, Marcon G, *et al.* Gold(III) complexes as potential antitumor agents: solution chemistry and cytotoxic properties of some selected gold(III) compounds. J Med Chem 2000; 43(19): 3541-8.
[http://dx.doi.org/10.1021/jm990492u] [PMID: 11000008]

[56] Gamberi T, Massai L, Magherini F, *et al.* Proteomic analysis of A2780/S ovarian cancer cell response to the cytotoxic organogold(III) compound Aubipy(c). J Proteomics 2014; 103: 103-20.
[http://dx.doi.org/10.1016/j.jprot.2014.03.032] [PMID: 24705091]

[57] Messori L, Cinellu MA, Merlino A. Protein Recognition of Gold-Based Drugs: 3D Structure of the Complex Formed When Lysozyme Reacts with Aubipy(c). ACS Med Chem Lett 2014; 5(10): 1110-3.
[http://dx.doi.org/10.1021/ml500231b] [PMID: 25313321]

[58] Petrović V, Petrović S, Joksić G, *et al.* Inhibition of Na(+)/K(+)-ATPase and cytotoxicity of a few selected gold(III) complexes. J Inorg Biochem 2014; 140: 228-35.
[http://dx.doi.org/10.1016/j.jinorgbio.2014.07.015] [PMID: 25173578]

[59] Colotti G, Ilari A, Fiorillo A, *et al.* Metal-based compounds as prospective antileishmanial agents: inhibition of trypanothione reductase by selected gold complexes. ChemMedChem 2013; 8(10): 1634-7.
[PMID: 24039168]

CHAPTER 6

Oral Delivery by Nanostructures for the Treatment of Cancer

Mahendar Porika[1], Rama Narsimha Reddy Anreddy[2,*], Radhika Tippani[1] and **Srividya Lonkala[2]**

[1] *Department of Biotechnology, Kakatiya University, Warangal, 506009, Telangana State, India*

[2] *Department of Pharmacology, Jyothishmathi Institute of Pharmaceutical Sciences, Ramakrishna Colony, Thimmapur, Karimnagar 505481, Telangana State, India*

Abstract: Oral administration of a drug is the most convenient route of treatment for the majority of diseases/disorders. However, there are limitations such as poor solubility, low intrinsic permeability, efflux transport, and extensive metabolism by the gastrointestinal (GI) tract/liver. To overcome these problems, nanoparticles (NPs) have been extensively studied as drug carriers. Previous results suggest that NP therapy can enhance the efficacy, while reducing side effects simultaneously. The development of nanotechnology for the management of cancer, a PEGgylated liposome NP formulation filled with anticancer drug (doxorubicin) had been developed as a first NP based therapy and received FDA approval in 1995. Approximately 20 varieties nanomedicine preparations are in for cancer chemotherapy clinical investigation. Various nano carriers used for cancer therapy need stabilization without effecting the physiological action of drug, its deposition at site of intended tumour and also decrease toxicity. The chapter emphases on NP technology with main focus on the formulation of nanomedicine for cancer therapy. This technique involves liposomes, polymeric NPs, polymeric conjugates, micelles, dendrimers, polymersomes and inorganic/metallic NPs.

Keywords: Cancer therapy, Intravenous, Nanoparticles, Nanomedicine, Oral drug administration, Treatment.

INTRODUCTION OF ORAL DRUG ADMINISTRATION

Oral administration is a route of drug administration where the drug is taken by mouth. It is a widely used route of administration in clinically. Also it is the most frequently used route of drug administration since it is most convenient, economic and painless. The mammalian intestinal inner layers are very absorptive also

---

*** Corresponding author Dr. Anreddy Rama Narsimha Reddy:** Professor of Pharmacology, Jyothishmathi Institute of Pharmaceutical Sciences, Beside LMD Police Station-505481, Ramakrishna Colony, Thimmapur, Karimnagar (Telangana State), India; Tel: +91 99084 57927; Email: anreddyram@gmail.com

Atta-ur-Rahman & M. Iqbal Choudhary (Eds.)

consists of microvilli which can even expand the 1 absorptive area in the gastrointestinal(GI) lumen to 300-400 m2 [1]. Intestinal cells (absorptive) and cup cells (bodily fluid emitting) spread the microvilli, having sprinkled with follicle associated epithelium (FAE). Tissues like lymphoid areas, Peyer's patches, secured with folded cells specifically detecting an antigen. M cells specialized for epithelium of mucosa-associated lymphoid tissues are critical in medication conveyance, because these are less ensured when taken up by body fluids [2, 3] and need more transcytotic limit [4]. Transcytosis is the vesicular transport of macromolecules from one side of a cell to the other. In spite of these potential favorable circumstances, oral delivery presents a few basic issues, especially for proteins: (i) poor steadiness in the stomach pH (ii) low bioavailability and (iii) fluid boundaries can also obstruct drug uptake affecting resulting ingestion. To overcome these restrictions, nanoparticle (NP) solutions are prepared in such a way that entire body and ensure a timely release in a controlled way. The NP surface area is adjusted to improve or decrease biological adhesion to target tumour cells. The barriers for the NPs to penetrate into the epithelial surfaces are mucus form layers protecting the epithelial layer surfaces [5 - 11].

Mucus is formed in our body professionally to protect surface layers of epithelial tissues by trapping pathogens, external particles and removing them rapidly. It is secreted to clear pathogens and also helpful in lubrication of the epithelium as and when materials passes through them, due to which NPs that fail to penetrate the upper layers of GIT decreasing their time of residence.

Role of Mucus in GIT

Mucus is composed of sugars, amino acids, peptides, lipids, salts, antibodies, bacteria and cellular debris. Mucin is a component of mucus made of protein, it is found free or bound to cells [6, 12]. The mucin monomers secreted will bind together by disulfide bonds to give a polymer [13]. It comprises of 2-5% of mucus net weight, mucin polymers bind forming cross-links forming dynamic viscoelastic gel in GIT required for protection and lubrication [14]. In GIT there exists always a constant turnover of adherent and glycocalyx layers constantly working on removal of organic debris and toxic substances entering through diet [15 - 17]. Hence a balanced mechanism exists between secretion of mucus and its removal degradation for maintenance of thickness of mucus layer. Stomach maintains pH of 1.5 to 7 over a mucus thickness of only about 200µm so always there raises a question of how food is able to digest in stomach region without being digesting itself, classical answer for this is only existence of dynamic protective mucosal secretions. Stomach degrades mucus and continuously maintains counterbalance of mucus secretion even at constant presence of low pH and digestive enzymes [13, 18]. The process of lubrication is an important protective mechanism of mucus in GIT. Mucus entraps biologically active substances which induce inflammation or healing processes after their release, like trefoil factors.

NANOTECHNOLOGY AND NANOMATERIALS

Nanotechnology is widely acknowledged as one of the main techniques of this century and accordingly huge advances have been made in with increased funds in global research on nanomaterials technologies [19]. A wide variety of nanoparticles are formulated and nanotechnology has evolved as main research area in the modern scientific era. The studies on NPs shows novel and varied properties differentiated from large scale unique applications. Nanotechnology is defined by size naturally varied on study of diverse fields including bio chemistry, molecular biology and immunology. Nanomaterials are nowadays widely attracted scientists because of their highly desirable properties [20]. NPs are structures of molecular sizes 1- 100 nm at least in one dimension. The word "nano" is prefixed commonly for particles of hundred nanometers in size. Optimized nanocarriers in terms of physical, chemical and biological properties are thereby absorbed by cells faster than particles of large size, for the effective treatment of many diseases [21] for successful delivery of bioactive substances available in the market. NPs are usually formulated as nanocapsules and nanospheres. The 3 uptake of orally delivered NPs by intestinal cells and its fate is determined by its size. NP surface properties direct the extent of NP uptake into the cells. Based on the nature of the drug to be encapsulated and of the polymers constituting the carrier various techniques are devised for preparation of NP.

NP surface properties are of utmost importance for their absorption by intestinal epithelial cells. Therefore, many approaches have been developed to increase mucosal uptake of NPs, by modifying their surface properties or by coupling a targeting molecule at their surface.

Surface properties can be modified by coating the NP surface with hydrophilic stabilizing, bio-adhesive polymers or surfactants or by incorporating hydrophilic biodegradable copolymers in the formulation. Modification of zeta potential, hydrophobicity, influences formulation of colloidal stability, protein adsorption and NP muco-adhesive properties at the surface, and ultimately oral absorption of the NPs. The main target of preparation these NP by addition of hydrophilic polymers like PEG (polyethylene glycol) or chitosan is to increase their passage across the intestinal mucosa *via* specific interactions between intestinal epithelium and nanocarriers [22]. Thus, modified NP's either by improving non-specific interactions with the cell apical surface or by grafting a specific ligand targeting epithelial intestinal cells ensure drug encapsulation in protective synthetic colloidal carriers to deliver drug in a pre-operated manner, for successful oral delivery of treating agents [23].

Nanotechnology is an important and ever growing field under medicine and pharmacy for developing drugs and drug delivery systems. Nanotechnology helps in designing and formulating medications with better therapeutic efficiency. NP based science helps in early detection and prevention, improved diagnosis, proper treatment and follow-up of complex diseases like cancer, diabetes, Parkinson's disease (PD), Alzheimer's disease (AD), cardiovascular diseases (CVD) as well as different kinds of serious inflammatory or infectious diseases [24]. In this present chapter, we highlighted the features of oral administration of drugs using nanotechnologies that are distinct from existing cancer therapies, and explains how these provide the potential for therapeutic effects that are not been achievable with other modalities. The outbreak of NP delivery systems is becoming increasingly recognized, with various examples of first generation nanoparticles approved by the FDA for treatment, and targeted nanocarriers in clinical phase development. Many nanocarrier delivery systems in clinical phase are highlighted in this chapter to demonstrate how these systems are translated to the clinic and the advantages they provide for the treatment of various diseases [20].

NPS FOR THE TREATMENT OF CANCER

Cancer

Cancer is a group of diseases characterized by the uncontrolled proliferation of body's abnormal cells with the potential to invade or spread to other parts of the body. All cancers are not malignant, few are benign and they do not spread to other regions of body. Physiological symptoms of one particular possible tumour in a majority of cases are i) an unusual lump or swelling anywhere in the body, ii) unexplained weight loss, iii) breathlessness, iv) new changes to a mole, v) persistent cough, vi)unusual bleeding from sides viz., rectum, vagina *etc.* vii) persistent indigestion and bowel changes, viii) difficulty if swallowing. These symptoms give evidence of cancer that may also occur due to other issues. About 100 different cancer types/entities affecting humans [25]. Cancer is one of the leading causes of death in the world. According to the 2014 World Cancer Report, nearly 14 million new cancer cases and 8.2 million cancer deaths were reported in 2012. Among the different types of cancer, lung cancer is associated with the greatest mortality (1.5 million deaths), then comes liver (745 000 deaths), stomach (723 000 deaths), colorectal (694 000 deaths), breast (521 000 deaths), and esophageal cancer (400 000 deaths) [26]. Number of new cancer cases are expected to increase by 70%, from 14 million to 22 million, in the next 2 decades [27]. Anticancer drugs are agents which aim to prevent the maturation and proliferation of neoplasms. Systemically applied drugs enter the bloodstream, distributed to all parts of the body and cause destruction of cancer cells by interfering with their ability to divide and grow. Many side effects associated with anticancer agents occur because these therapies destroy the normal cells in addition to cancerous cells. The harmful effects of anticancer drugs include bone marrow suppression, vomiting, alopecia, pain and nerve changes, changes in fertility and sexuality, anaemia, damage to vital organs like kidney and liver etc. The classification of anticancer agents which are used for the treatment of many types of cancer are summarized in Table **1**.

Table 1. Classification of Antineoplastic Agents / Anticancer Drugs.

1	*Alkylating Agents*	• Nitrogen mustards: Melphalan, Cyclophosphamide, Ifosfamide • Nitrosoureas • Alkylsulfonates • Ethyleneimines • Triazene • Methyl Hydrazines • Platinum Coordination complexes: Cisplatin, Carboplatin, Oxaliplatin
2	*Antimetabolites*	• Folate Antagonists: Methotrexate • Purine antagonists • Pyrimidine antagonists: 5-Fluorouracil, Cytarabibe
3	*Plant Products*	• Vinca Alkaloids: Vincristine, Vinblastine • Taxanes: Paclitaxel, Docetaxel • Epipodophyllotoxins: Etoposide • Camptothecins: Irinotecan
4	*Antitumour Antibiotics (Anthracyclines)*	• Doxorubicin, Bleomycin
5	*Miscellaneous*	• Hydroxyurea • Imatinib Mesylate • Rituximab • Epirubicin • Bortezomib • Zoledronic Acid • Geftinib • Leucovorin • Pamidronate • Gemcitabin • L-Asparaginase

(Table 1) contd.....

6	**Hormones and Antagonists**	• Corticosteroids: Prednisone, Dexamethasone • Estrogens: Ethinyloestradiol • Antiestrogens: Tamoxifen • Progesteron derivative: Megestrol Acetate • Androgen: Testosterone propionate • Antiandrogen: Flutamide, Bicalutamide • Aromatase inhibitor: Letrozole, Anastrazole • 5-alpha reductase inhibitor: Finasteride • GnRH Analogue: Leuprolide, Buserelin • Growth Hormone, glucagon and insulin inhibitor: Octreotide

The use of anticancer drugs likes methotrexate, cisplatin, cyclophosphamide, tamoxifen and doxorubicin is generally based on the treatment strategy and location of the tumour [25]. Antitumour drugs are not only used directly in all different types of cancers but within conjunction with surgery, radiotherapy and immunotherapy in the combined modality approach for many solid tumours, especially malignant or metastatic cancers.

Many cancer drugs are molecules of minute sizes which are being ingested orally or injected, diffuse through vascular spaces in the blood and diffuse in the matrix to reach solid tumours. Combination of drugs used in therapy is complex and have larger drug delivery mechanism. The molecular size exactly required to travel through vascular pores from blood stream to get the tumour site is not fully understood. The size limitation may be < 20 nm.

Nanotechnology is farther more developed for the management of diabetes at a rapid pace owing to its adaptation from success in treatments for other diseases like cancer, for which the first NP based therapy, a PEGylated liposome NP formulation loaded with the chemotherapeutic drug doxorubicin, received FDA approval in 1995.

20 different nanomedicine formulations or even more are currently under clinical investigation for cancer therapy. The ideal nanocarrier for drug delivery and cancer chemotherapy should

 i. Maintain the stability of drug without changing the pharmacological activity.
 ii. Should not be easily metabolized by systemic circulation before reaching a particular level in the blood required to act on the tumour site.
 iii. Concentrate and reach at the particular site of tumour.
 iv. Should have a lesser toxicity when compared to that of free drug.

Other important features include characteristic appearance on MRI for evaluation by molecular imaging and thus guiding chemotherapy. In general, regimens dependent on schedule requires steady state drug levels ideal for controlled drug delivery systems (CDDSs) [28]. Such CDDSs overcome the problems encountered with administration of cytotoxic agents systemically as these drugs lack specificity and cause significant damage to noncancerous tissues (systemic toxicity). So when cytotoxic drugs are given systemically there are issues due to lack of specificity of the drug towards cancer tissue and hence they damage noncancerous tissue, bone marrow, hair follicles, intestinal epithelium leading to systemic toxicity, anemia, immune suppression and alopecia.

In addition to lack of specificity and cytotoxicity the effects of the drugs are further increased with escalation in dosage required for solid cancers. Since these chemotherapeutic agents have low therapeutic index and rapid excretion rate [29]. When a nanocarrier is added it acts by prolonging the half-life of drug thus improving the pharmacokinetics. Also nanocarriers improve the aqueous solubility of poorly soluble anti-cancer drugs thus reducing the cytotoxicity by removing the cytotoxic agent which are mainly solvents like Cremophor EL which are widely used as dissolving agent [30]. The more relevant advantages of nanocarriers as CDDS over free drugs are summarized as follows:

Goals of targeted nanoscale drug delivery systems.

- The drug should be nontoxic and Biocompatible and biodegradable.
- It should improve cellular absorption of the drug and intra cellular transfer.
- Should concentrate the drug at the tumour site within required time period.
- Protect the drug from degradation and from premature clearance.
- Reduce the drug leakage during the transit time to reach the target site.
- Minimal drug localization in the sensitive and vital tissue (non-target).
- Improve drug localization in the tumour by
    a. Passive targeting
    b. Active targeting

Here, we highlight the various NP technologies (Fig. **1** and **2**), with main emphasis on the formulation of nanocarrier drug delivery systems for cancer chemotherapy.

Nanomedicine is the use of nanotechnology in the field of medicine. Nanomedicine is expected to help us to reach the goals of targeted drug delivery systems. Years of research and development has led us to the path of nanomedicine where the results are promising [32 - 36]. As shown in Fig. (**1** and **2**), the NPs used for drug delivery can be readily fabricated from either soft (organic and polymeric) or hard (inorganic) materials, with their sizes being controlled typically in the range of 1-100 nm and particles/ structures being engineered to pack anticancer drugs in a variety of configurations [37, 38].

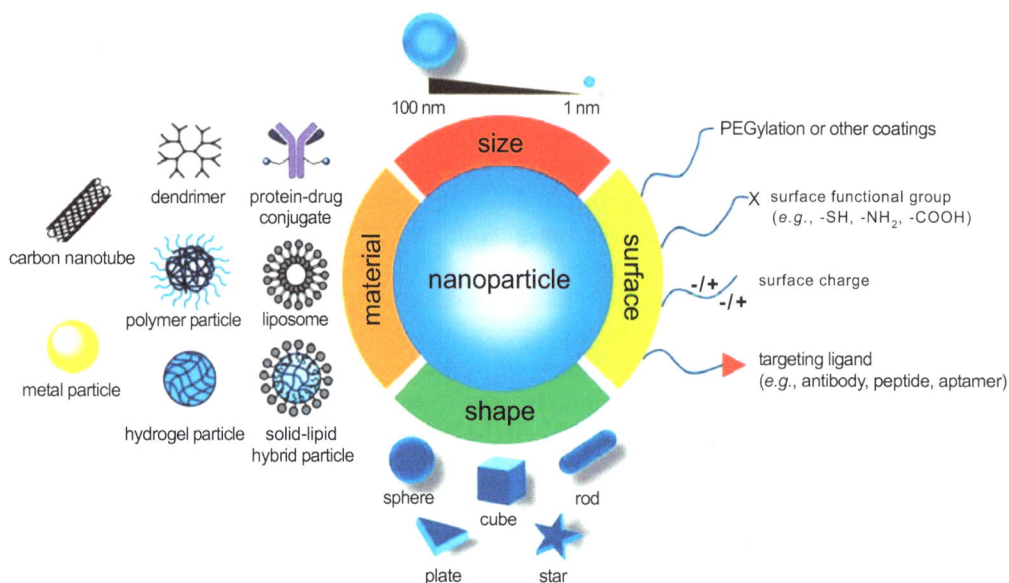

Fig. (1). A summary of NPs that have been explained here with NP as carriers for drug delivery in cancer treatment, together with illustrations on biological, physical and chemical characteristics [31].

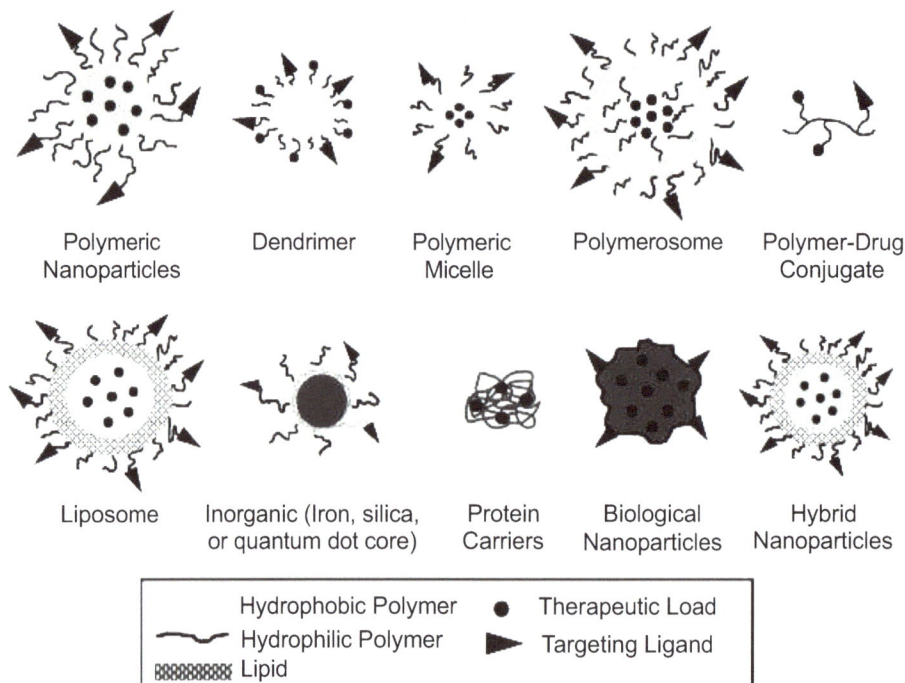

Fig. (2). Various NPs used for the drug delivery NP technologies [39].

Compared to current traditional chemotherapy drugs, the delivery of anticancer drugs through a NP based platform offers many advantages, including:

i. Facilitation of drug absorption of the drugs which have low water solubility and concentration of the drug at the target sites in higher dosage.

ii. To save guard the drug from gastric and intestinal pH and digestive enzymes, so that the plasma half-life of the drug can be extended so has to reach at the target site.

iii. To evolve tissue or cell particular target drug so that improving the efficiency and minimizing the side effects (systemic).

iv. Systematic drug delivery system can be developed by releasing the drug in a controlled manner so as to dispense the drug in response to stimulus over a period of time (demonstrated as stimuli- responsive system).

v. Delivery of combination of different types of drugs and diagnostic agents simultaneously to improve the treatment outcome and escape multidrug resistance [36, 40, 41].

Nanocarriers For Cancer Treatment

In 1960s the first nanoscale drug delivery systems were first vesicles loaded with lipid, and later they became liposomes. The first controlled-release polymer systems for the delivery of macromolecules were explained in the year 1976 [42]. The modification of liposomes on surface and polymeric NPs with PEG) lead to increases in circulation time, or "stealth" properties [43, 44]. The development culminated in the approval of Doxil, a vesicle delivery system encapsulating the drug doxorubicin has proven to be a potential for treating various kinds of cancer [45, 46]. Following after that tremendous progress was observed in the development of engineered NPs that have multifunctional abilities and also "smart" properties such as the sensitivity to the environmental conditions to facilitate more efficient drug delivery systems. Presently, more than 70 clinical trials evaluated reports on NP carriers, 208 drug conjugates 10 evaluations, and 361 vesicle-based carriers evaluations [47] are available. The trials include combinational treatments using various routes of administration, like oral pulmonary. Other NP technologies for cancer chemotherapy constitute polymeric NPs [48, 49], liposomes [50, 51], micelles [52 - 54], dendrimers [55, 56], polymer conjugates [57] and inorganic NPs [58, 59]. The diversity of delivery systems allows the NPs to be prepared with a divergent array of shapes, sizes and constitutions that enables new ones to be tailored for special applications. Although, the primary consideration while preparation of any drug delivery system is to achieve more effective treatment by controlling the drug concentration in the therapeutic window with lower side effects and also to improve patient acceptance (Fig. **3**). These treatment cycles allows effective maintenance reducing damage to normal cells and minimizes the recovery period.

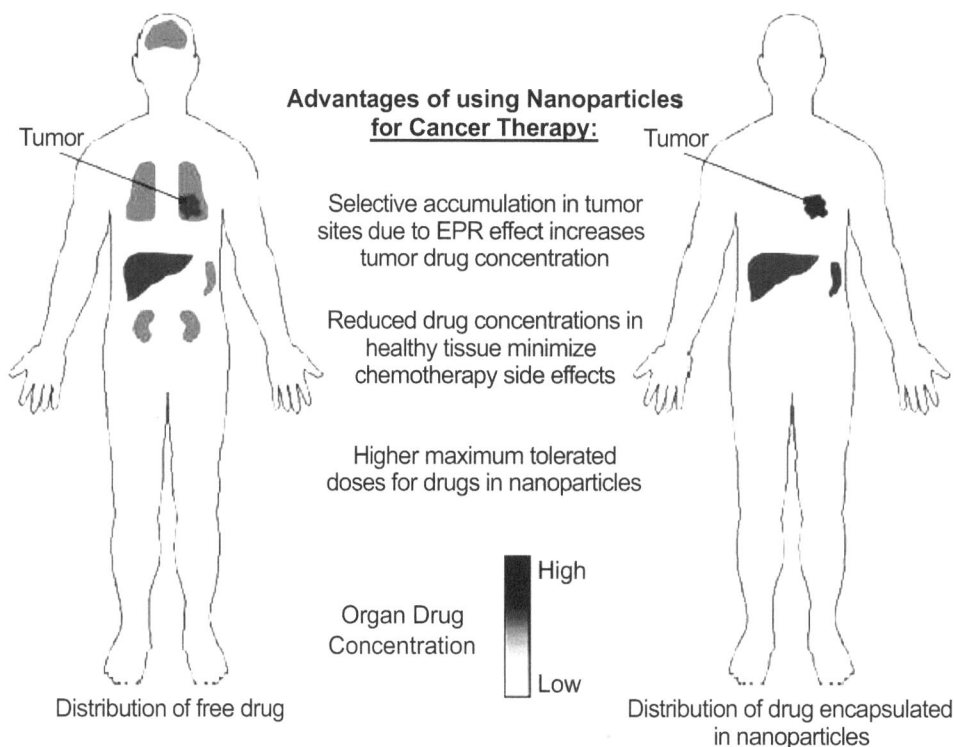

Advantages of using Nanoparticles for Cancer Therapy:

Selective accumulation in tumor sites due to EPR effect increases tumor drug concentration

Reduced drug concentrations in healthy tissue minimize chemotherapy side effects

Higher maximum tolerated doses for drugs in nanoparticles

Organ Drug Concentration

High

Low

Distribution of free drug

Distribution of drug encapsulated in nanoparticles

Tumor

Tumor

Fig. (3). Advantages of using NPs as drug delivery system for cancer therapy over usage of free drugs [39].

Liposome NPs

Liposomes are phospholipid bilayer enclosing a vesicle which can be used as a drug carrier. They are list toxic suitable with acceptable biodegradation profile. Liposomes are suitable for the delivering drugs which are hydrophilic and hydrophobic in nature [60, 61]. They are stable because of encapsulation and give a controlled release and local action. Drugs can be loaded in liposomes achieved by i) formation of liposome in aqueous solution with a soluble drug ii) with the use of solvents (organic) iii) using lipophilic drugs iv) pH gradiation [62]. The factors effecting the releasing of the drug are solvent, pH, temperature, enzymes, volume *etc*. The lipid bilayer fuses with the bilayer of the cell membrane to dispense the drug (Fig. **4**). Usually, liposomes are 400 nm in size. Thus are rapidly cleared by monolayer phagocytic system. To avoid this rapid clearance, a process called PEGylation was developed in 1960; as biocompatible polymer, poly (ethylene glycol) (PEG; [CH2CH2O]n) that can be conjugated to the drug carrier [63]. The coating significantly increases the half-life of the drug. There are three generation of liposomes

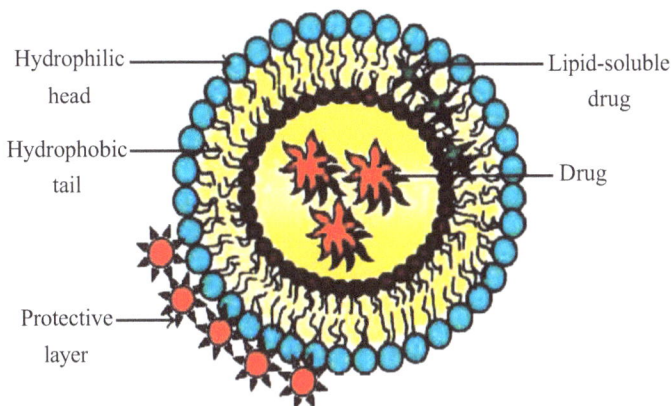

Fig. (4). Diagram of bi-layered membrane structure.

i. First generation- Naked liposomes with no modification on phospholipid surface.

ii. Second generation -Stealth liposome with a coating of PEG on the surface of vesicles.

iii. Third generation- Liposomes with incorporated surface ligands which improve the therapeutic index of the drug (by increasing the selectivity and specificity).

Liposomal formulations that are available on the market and in clinical trials are summarized in Table **2**.

Table 2. Liposomal formulations that are available on the market and in clinical trials [64].

Composition	Trade Name	Company	Indication	Administration
Liposomal daunorubicin	DaunoXome	Gilead Science	Kaposi's sarcoma	Intravenous
Stealth loposomal	Doxil/Caelyx	Ortho Biotech	Kaposi's sarcoma; refractory ovarian	Intramuscular
Doxorubicin		Schering-Plough	Cancer; refractory breast cancer	Intravenous
Liposomal doxorubicin	Myocet	Zeneus	Metastatic breast cancer in combination	Intravenous
			with cylophosphamide	

Composition	Trade Name	Company	Indication	Administration
Liposomal muramyl Tripeptide phosphatidyl Ethanolamine	MEPACT	Taked	Osteosarcoma	Intravenous
Cytarabine	Depocyt	SkyePharma PLC	Lymphomatous meningitis	Intrathecal
Liposomal vincristine	Onco-TCS	Inex Enzon	Non-hodgking lymphoma	Intravenous

The internal core entraps a hydrophilic drug, while lipid soluble drugs are entrapped between the hydrophobic tails of the phospholipids. The outer surface can be functionalized with PEG and ligands for active targeting [64]. The Fig. (**5**) explained about the drug delivery by the liposomes into the target tissues.

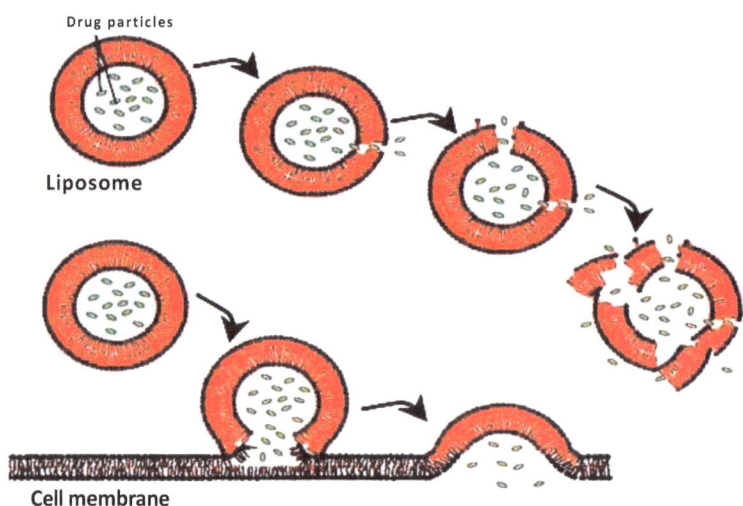

Fig. (5). Drug delivery by liposomes into the target tissue(s) [21].

Polymeric NPs

Polymeric NPs form the most effective nanocarriers for prolonged drug delivery and effective disease treatment. Lipid polymer hybrid NPs are polymeric NPs enveloped by a lipid layer that combines the highly biocompatible nature of lipids with structural integrity contributed by polymeric NPs. Drugs used in cancer therapy made from easy degradable polymers are an attractive option as good Drug delivery devices.

Polymeric NP are solid colloidal particles ranging from 10 to 1000 nm in diameter. They are of two varieties mainly nanocapsules and nanospheres. Drugs can be dissolved entrapped, encapsulated or attached to the NP matrix, it can also be covalently link to the polymer by means of an ester or amide bond which can be hydrolyzed easily by simple change in pH (Fig. **6**). These systems have wide surface areas drugs can also be adsorbed on their surface. They carry drugs to target cells and organs. The size promotes effective permission through cell membrane and allow them to remain stable in the blood.

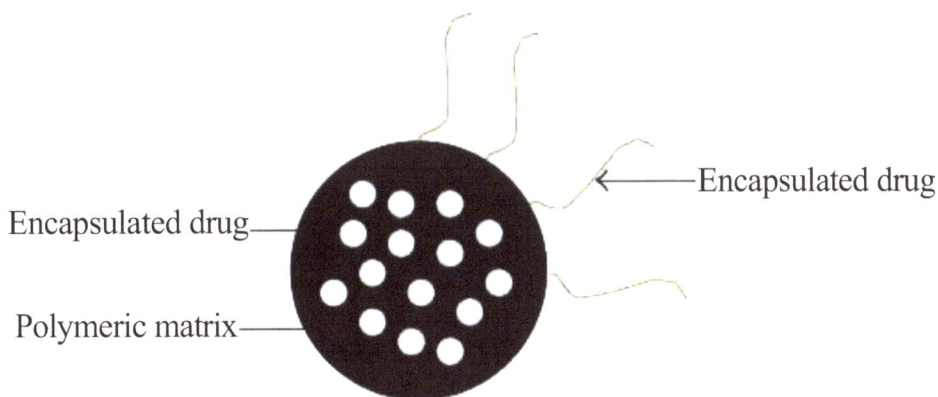

Fig. (6). A schematic representation of a polymeric nanoparticle as drug carriers: the drug is entrapped in the polymeric matrix and functional moieties lead to active targeting [64].

Both *in vitro* and *in vivo* multiple reports using polymer-based materials for drug delivery were made on polyalkylcyanoacrylate-based NPs releasing doxorubicin in 1980s [65]. Recently, the controlled release of various polymer carriers with drug attached by both covalent and non-covalent pathways allowed for the development of drug delivery system for cancer therapy and opened new lines for the delivery of polymers for the cancer therapy was reviewed by Ulbrich *et al.* [66]. Polymeric NPs provide significant flexibility during design because polymers can be biodegradable or non- biodegradable, and can be made synthetically or be derived from natural sources. Poly lactic acid (PLA), dextran, and chitosan are a few examples for the commonly used polymers for NP formation.

Biodegradable polymers consist of single monomers which act as subunit. After biodegradation these monomers are metabolized by normal metabolic pathways. The metabolism is controlled by properties of polymer like molecular weight, hydrophobicity, crystallinity; thus modifying drug release kinetics. To control the release of the drug and diffusion, the NP surface is stabilized by grafting, conjugating and adsorbing these polymers like PEG on to the surface. Thus creating a controlled manner of drug release which is not easily metabolized by the liver, hence increasing its half-life [67]. Table **3** explains the status of a few polymeric NPs in different stages of clinical trials which were developed for cancer therapy.

Table 3. Polymeric NPs in clinical trials [64].

Compound	Name	Status	Indication
Albumin-paclitaxel	Abraxane	Approved	Metastatic breast cancer
Doxorubicin	Transdrug	Approved	Hepatocarcinoma
Paclitaxel	Nanoxel	Phase I	Advanced breast cancer
Paclitaxel	Paclimer	Phase I	Various

Polymer-Drug Conjugate NPs

The nano-carrier type which is more explored are polymer drug conjugates of size <20 nm. They are formed by side chain grafting of drugs to polymer chains and are capable of delivering high doses of chemotherapy drugs. The first synthetic polymer HPMA-doxorubicin (N- (2-hydroxypropyl) methacrylamide) copolymer (PK1) was an anticancer drug conjugate to enter clinical trials for advanced breast cancer which is still ongoing in women [68]. Taking the example of drug Prolindac (AP5346) formed by a HMPA back bone copolymer with platinum grafted to the side chains *via* a pH sensitive chelator design to release the drug in the tumour tissue [69]. Preclinical data clearly shows the high efficacy for polymer-drug conjugates using multiple cancer models including a M5076 sarcoma platinum-resistant tumour xenograft mice model, multiple colon xenograft models, L1210 leukemia, and 0157 hybridoma models [70]. Oxaliplatin drug packed was ~10% (w/w) using a polymer chain of 25 kDa and the drug release was slow and delayed. Formulations were given intravenous once a week for three weeks and the polymer-drug conjugates significantly decreased tumour growth over one month due to more intracellular concentration of Platinum (Pt).

Polyamino acids side chains grafted with drugs on side chains instead of polymer drug, these conjugation led to high drug loading and efficacy [71, 72]. For example, polyglutamate-glycine-campthotecin conjugates (CT-2106) allowed the drug to load from 5 to 50%, adding a glycine linker drug load was found three fold over the normal range due to reduced steric hindrance. In clinical trials the drug load of 30% was used and trials were conducted for the stability and efficacy on human tumour xenograft mouse models [73]. The clinical trials conducted for the drug *i.e* polymer- drug conjugate (polyglutamate-paclitaxel) for cancer therapies showed 20 -40% of drug load allowed. These trials were conducted for the treatment of multiple cancers like prostate cancer, neck cancer, metastatic colorectal cancer and metastatic breast cancer (Phase III). In The drug Xyotax,

Paclitaxel is grafted to polyglutamic acid (30-40 kDa) forming a polymer drug conjugate [74]. The patients treated with Xyotax had a better median survival time than control group; overall survival was unaltered. So the benefit was reduction of side effects like neurotoxicity [75].

Thus we infer that optimal formulation requires more development and also polymer drug conjugation might help the efficiency of drug by improving the load and tissue distribution. The resulting formulation could also be considered a new molecular entity, complicating regulatory approval.

Micelle NPs

Polymeric micelles are nano-carrier drugs of usual size which are able to overcome the limitations of oral delivery and has good bioavailability when given orally. They are considered as ideal because of their modifiable properties and the high drug loading capacity. The usually comprise of a core shell structure constituted by amphiphilic block copolymers. The copolymer consists of more than to polymeric chains exhibiting different hydrophobicity. The hydrophobic segments make the hydrophobic inner core and thus are protected from the environmental exposure. Whereas the hydrophilic chains form the outer shell stabilizing the core (Fig. **7**).

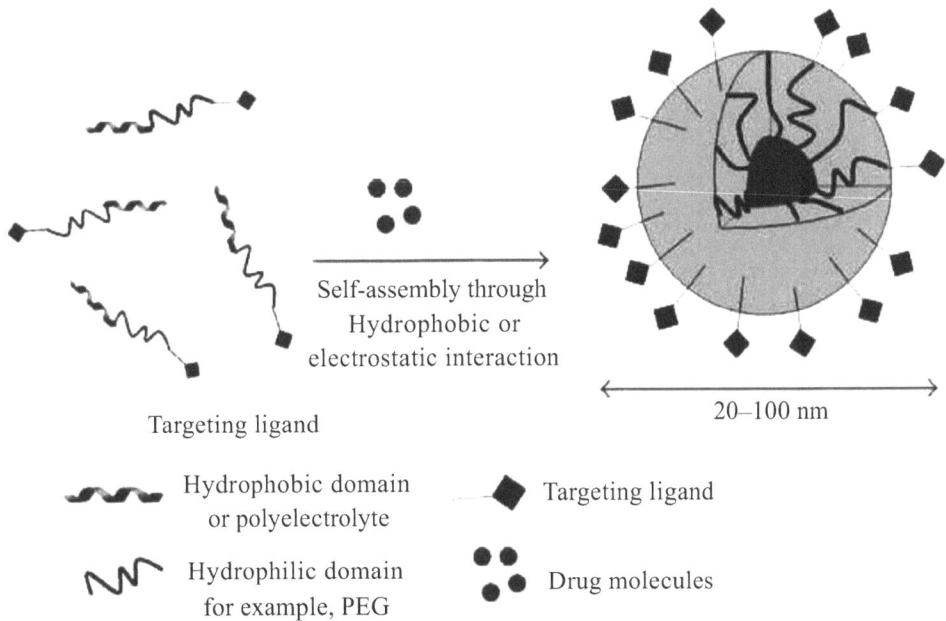

Fig. (7). Polymeric micelle core-shell structure and drug encapsulation [76].

Hence they are best for oral delivery of drugs. They provide maximal drug absorption by muco-adhesion, protection of the loaded drug from GI environment and releasing the drug in a controlled manner [76]. Also the hydrophobic drugs which are given intravenously only by adding adjuvants like ethanol or Cremophor EL which have toxic side effects can effectively be given without any adjuvant directly after incorporation of drug into micelles. Since the outer hydrophilic shell provides the protection and releases the drug in regulated manner, combination of two or more therapeutic agents can be given in this manner. Since these micelles are biodegradable the drug release can be achieved by erosion of polymers or by diffusion of the drug through polymer matrix following polymer swelling. Also change in pH, temperature causes drug release. Specific target delivery can be done by modifying the surface of the micelles using ligands like anti bodies, peptides and small molecules. So the systemic toxicity is reduced and efficacy of the drug is improved [76].

Micelles are ideal for delivering hydrophobic drugs [77]. The micelle drug Genexol-PM is under clinical evaluation [78], NK911 and NC- 6004 [79, 80]. It was earlier given approval for treatment of non-targeted cancer therapy, later it was approved for primary therapy in treatment of metastatic breast cancer and non-small cell lung cancer. Phase II trials now being conducted for metastatic, pancreatic cancer treatment is USA. Genexol-PM is a biodegradable micelles of size ~60 nm comprising of a block copolymer poly (D,L-lactide) (PDLLA) (1.75 kDa)-mPEG (2 kDa) and paclitaxel. It releases paclitaxel in controlled form. So it is better tolerated than up to three times than Taxol (60 mg kg 1 *vs.* 20 mg kg 1, respectively). In studies on Sprague- Dawley rats it proved to that the tolerated dose (LD50) was nearly 20 fold more than Taxol. Paclitaxel shows an affinity towards liver and tumour tissue, hence the drug gets accumulated here leads to tumour cytotoxicity and tumour destruction thus reducing the tumour volume [81]. In addition, recently Krishnamurthy *et al.* [82] also reported that Phenformin-loaded polymeric micelles are targeted to both cancer cells and cancer stem cells *in vitro* and *in vivo* and results in the prevention of relapse and metastasis. The polymeric micelles under clinical trials are showed in Table **4**.

Table 4. Polymeric micelles in clinical trials [83].

Polymeric Micelle	Block Copolymer	Drug	Diameter	Indication	Clinical Phase
NK012	PEG-PGIu(SN-38)	SN-38	20 nm	Breast cancer	II
NK105	PEG-P(aspartate)	Paditaxel	85 nm	Advanced stomach cancer	II

(Table 4) contd.....

Polymeric Micelle	Block Copolymer	Drug	Diameter	Indication	Clinical Phase
SP1049C	Pluronic L61 and FI27	Doxorubicin	22-27 nm	Adenocarcinoma of oesophagus, gastroesophageal junction and stomach	III
NC-6004	PEG-PGIu(cisplatin)	Cisplatin	30 nm	Solid tumors	I/II
Genexol-PM	PEG-P(D,L-lactide)	Paditaxel	20-50 nm	Breast cancer	IV
				Pancreatic cancer	II
				Non-small-cell lung cancer in combination with carboplatin	II
				Pancreatic cancer in combination with gemcitabine	I/II
				Ovarian cancer in combination with carboplatin	I/II

Polymersome NPs

Polymersomes are similar to that of liposomes in structure, but are made of synthetic polypeptide/ polymer amphiphilic and self- assembling to form shell polymer vesicles (~100 nm) when hydrated and extruded. Discher *et al* [84] described vesicles which were consisted of amphiphilic diblock copolymers with less aqueous penetrability. So these synthetic block copolymers have radii ranging from 50 nm to 5µM with their basic shape alternating between spherical or cylindrical which is mainly dependent on the hydrophilicity/hydrophobicity ratio. The membrane core thickness depends on the diblock copolymer (molecular weight). The synthetic copolymer which forms the core enables to manipulate the features of the membrane and controls the permeability drug release and stability of polymersome. When the polymer chain disrupts, destabilizes or degrades the drug is released which is in a controlled manner. Blood plasma incubation studies of polymersomes exhibited the adherence and uptake by white blood cells within time period of 10 h. In a study Polymersomes packed with paclitaxel and doxorubicin showed a therapeutic efficacy on breast cancer tumour xenograft model after a single intravenous (*i.v.*) injection at the maximum tolerated dose (2.5 mg /kg for each drug). The tumor size was reduced within five days post injection in contrast to the control groups [85].

Protein NPs

Protein nanoparticles are biodegradable carriers which are non-antigenic in which the drugs are incorporated. Albumin is the main protein used for fabrication of protein NP (~130 nm). So albumin accumulates in solid tumours and is non-immunogenic so it can be used as targeted delivery for anti-tumour drugs. Albumin-bound paclitaxel (Abraxane, ABI-008) has been approved by US FDA in the treatment of breast cancer and other types of cancers [86]. When compared to taxols which exhibits limited ADME (absorption, distribution, metabolism, and excretion) properties and hypersensitivity, albumin bound paclitaxel is superior because of less side effects as it is a hydrophobic drug. Preclinical studies reveal that the bound paclitaxel concentration to albumin in endothelial cells and in the extravascular space was significantly raised (3-10 fold) [87, 88]. It was identified that albumin may show intrinsic targeting ability to tumour site, which is also supported by the increased permeability and retention (EPR) effect that may play an additional role in tumour growth. Among all, the albumin-bound paclitaxel formulation allows larger dosages than the Taxol formulation (260 mg m 2 *vs.* 175 mg m 2, respectively) and improved efficacy and safety [87]. Albumin is now studied for delivery of molecules which have reduced water solubility like rapamycin (~2.5 mg/ml). The result have been promising so albumin-bound rapamycin (ABI-009) is under clinical phase trial for the treatment of non-hematologic tumours.

Dendrimer NPs

Dendrimers is the word is derived from Greek word Dendron meaning tree owing to its structure of branching which appears like a tree usually of size ranging from 1-15 nm. They are circular highly branched three dimensional synthetic macromolecules which have adjustable shape and size. They comprise of many branches in which the terminal branches are active also known as generations. These generations arrive from an initiator main core known as generation zero. The chemotherapeutic agents and drug molecules are attached to the large surface area is provided by the branches of dendrimers by covalent conjugation or electrostatic adsorption. So the agent is trapped into the cavities of the core regions *via* hydrogen bonding or hydrophobic interaction [76]. Dendrimers have significant molecular monodispersity and controlled ADME for systemic drug delivery with easily degradable chemical bonding for drug dissociation [89].

Amphiphilic dendrimers can form micelles by self-assembling with hydrophilic groups on the surface of functional group. Drug pharmacokinetic release profile is maintained through the nature of polymer chain, which is designed for the release of a payload.

The most widely studied dendrimers are a group belonging to the family of PAMAM (polyamidoamine) dendrimers. These show great potential for drug delivery since these polymers are biodegradable and biocompatible with more aqueous solubility [90]. Recently, a G5-PAMAM dendrimer has been developed with a diameter of 5nm and more than 100 functional amines on the surface. This nanocarrier was developed for the delivery of methotrexate in under preclinical studies. The dendrimer surface charge is introduced by changing amines at terminal end by acetyl groups. So that, the G5-PAMAM dendrimer can conjugate with methotrexate (as the cytotoxic agent) and also with folate as the targeting molecule. The systemic distribution of drug in mice for subcutaneous tumours showed intracellular accumulation and internalization of dendrimers in human xenograft KB tumours that had excessive folate receptors. Under *in vivo* delivery of the G5-PAMAM dendrimer conjugated with methotrexate induced a 10 fold decrease in size of tumour when viewed against intravenous administration of free methotrexate at the same concentration(in moles) [91]. The study provides the basis for further preclinical studies on dendrimers, which are now study for cancer chemotherapy.

Myc *et al* [92] have developed "avidimers". These dendrimers are used for targeted drug delivery by detecting the vasculature of tumours by using methotrexate-PAMAM bioconjugate platform functionalized with small targeting ligands [93]. Non-targeted and folate-targeted G5-PAMAM dendrimers differentially accumulated into a human KB cell line xenograft tumour model within a day (8%- 10% targeted *versus* 2% non-targeted I.D./g of tissues) [91].

The more the accumulation of drug at tumour site results in more reduction of tumour growth, minimal toxicity, and higher survival time when compared to free drug at equal molar concentration. More important is the current efficacy studies on targeted transferrin- cyclodextrin-siRNA NPs (CALAA-01, ~70 nm) in animal models of human epithelial cancer which resulted in significant reduction of tumour size and tumour differential distribution [94, 95].

Inorganic NPs

Many inorganic NPs are primarily metal-based and described as good anticancer agents. The main cytotoxicity of NPs like zinc oxide is due to the release of metal (zinc) ions that are dissolved intracellularly, that follows induction of reactive oxygen species (ROS). This phenomenon causes disequilibrium of metal - mediated protein activity and oxidative stress, eventually leads to death the cell. Soluble extracellular metal shows minute cellular toxicity. The ongoing research reveals that extracellular soluble zinc, when exposed to culture and phosphate media, leads to formation of poorly soluble amorphous zinc- carbonate phosphate Ppt (precipitates). This Ppt is supposed to protect the cell from the cytotoxicity of zinc [96].

As showed in Fig. (**8**), all Zn oxide (ZnO) NPs are actively taken by cell endocytosis. Some NPs enter the cell rapidly, while others pass through phagocytosis and pinocytosis bound to endosomes and lysosomes. At low pH, the ZnO NPs, dissolution rate is rapid, which causes lysosome destabilization. The pH of first endosomes is relatively low, *i.e.*, 6.3, that favors the release of zinc ions which are soluble. It decreases further to pH 5.5 at next endosomes and pH 4.7 in lysosomes, where a rapid solubility rate of ZnO NPs is found causing lysosome instability. These show that at low pH necessary for the release of zinc ions into blood or extracellular fluid, which has a normal pH of 7, is not favorable. This process causes an improvement in release of soluble zinc ions in the cell. The increase in intracellular zinc concentration leads to zinc-dependent protein activity disequilibrium, finally resulting in cytotoxicity. Increase in zinc ions increases ROS concentration, causing cytotoxicity of cells by oxidative stress [97]. In a Clinical trial conducted on brain and recurrent prostate cancer in Germany Aminosilane coated Iron oxide NPs (Nanotherm M01) is under phase II in conjunction with hyperthermia and thermoablation. Phase I evaluation study revealed that prostate tumor cells could be destroyed by magnetic iron oxide NP [99]. Current investigation silica NPs coated with gold nanoparticles is a pilot study for head and neck cancer therapy which is similar to the magnetic iron oxide that absorb near-infrared laser energy and causes conversion of light energy to heat energy for killing solid tumours.

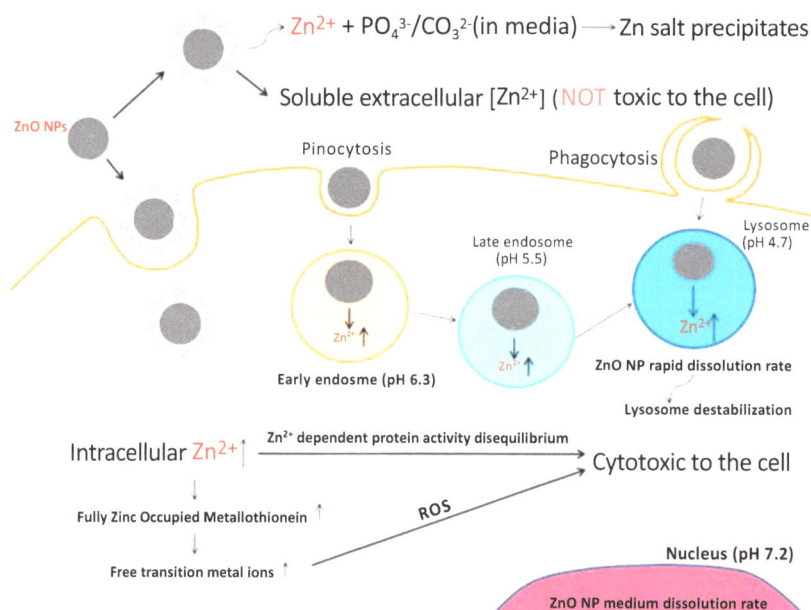

Fig. (8). The mechanism of the cytotoxicity of ZnO NPs [98]. Abbreviations: NP, nanoparticle; ZnO, zinc oxide.

Similarly, titanium dioxide [100] and cerium oxide [101] are reported as anticancer agents by evaluating them in a wide range of tumour cells. As shown in Fig. (**9**), NPs induce oxidative stress by producing ROS which can cause lysosomal damage, necrosis and caspase mediated apoptosis.

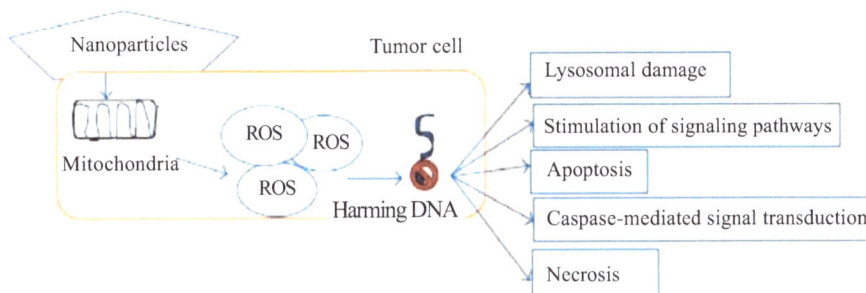

Fig. (9). The mechanism of apoptosis and necrosis mediated by NPs in tumour cells [102].

Healthy tissues have non-specific accumulation of drugs that provides a concern for NP drug delivery systems. The principle is applied local sensitization through light or temperature that may reduce overall toxicity, but this may damage adjacent tissues as well. Eventually, inorganic nanoparticles may not provide more advantages over other types of NPs for systemic targeting of cancer cells since they are not biodegradable, have low payloads, and does not contain any controlled release properties.

STRATEGIES FOR CANCER THERAPY USING NPS

Metastatic Cancer

The dissemination of primary tumour cells to distant organs or sites is called metastasis. Detachment of cancer cells occurs from the primary tumour site and enters the blood circulation and this follows cancer cells to attach to other organs such as the lungs, liver, kidneys, brain, colon, lymph nodes, skin, and bones, where they can invade and proliferate [103, 104]. Despite of their significant increase in the understanding of metastatic cancer pathogenesis, early diagnosis, surgical methods, and irradiation treatment, most cancer deaths are due to metastases that are difficult to treat. The main reasons include resistance to treatments, difficulty to access the tumour sites and removal of all cancer cells after surgery, or physiological barriers for drug access such as the blood-brain barrier (BBB). Hence, developing the effective treatment of metastatic cancer is a difficult still, even though various treatment modalities are approved and are in clinical study. Owing to knowledge regarding tumour biology its microenvironment, signaling pathways and metastatic study the cancer treatment has advanced to a greater stage. Drugs are now being developed against a wide range of targets that include transferase inhibitors, angiogenesis inhibitors, matrix metalloproteinase inhibitors, epidermal growth-factor receptor inhibitors, and migration inhibitors [105]. To avoid drug resistance during cancer treatment combination of the drugs are used maximizing the benefit reducing the side effects [106]. NP delivery system provides these benefits. The drug distribution along with NP had a higher concentration of drug at tumour site in contrast to free drug in both targeted and non-targeted delivery system. Multiple drugs can be loaded together in single NP with regulating the release of each drug enhancing patient tolerance when compared to complex to multi drug treatments.

Non-targeted NPs

Non-targeted NPs which are flow in the blood showing significant bioavailability and drug accumulation at tumour site by enhanced permeability and retention effect (EPR) (Fig. **10**).

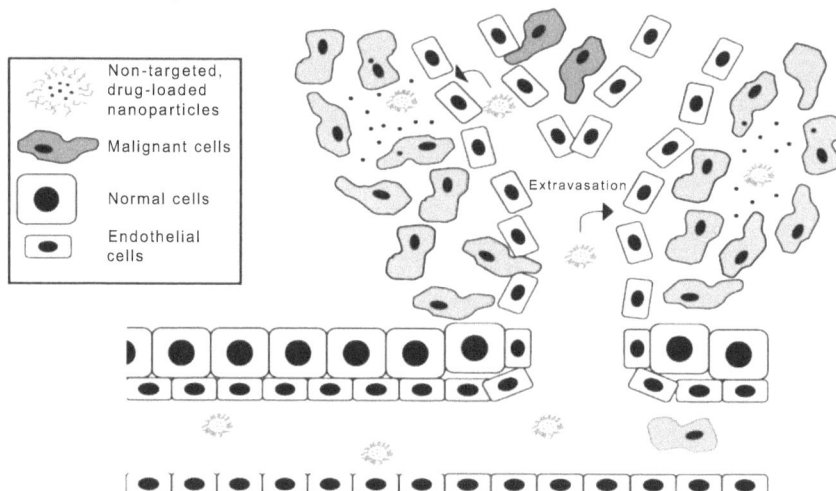

Fig. (10). Schematic diagram of passive targeting of NPs *via* an enhanced permeability and retention effect. The smaller the size of NPs more is the circulation for more time period, accumulate and extravasate into tumour site through leaky tumour vasculature [39].

The EPR effect allows targeting of NPs to tumours passively due to histopathological abnormalities in the tumour vascular system [107, 108]. Inter-endothelial gap defects increase the vascular permeability in tumours, allowing extrusion of NPs up to 400 nm [109]. Since the lymphatic drainage of tumour is poor the NP are more accumulated at the tumour site helping in the release of the drug. The nano-carriers release the drug locally in the extravascular space improving the drug concentration in the tumour the hydrophobic drugs are the ones which are released extracellularly, diffuse and accumulate at tumour site taken up by cancer cells destroying the tumour. In tumour populations- cell density, microenvironment, antigen expression and vasculature density are significantly differ among different types of cancers and also within primary and secondary metastatic sites.

Therefore, NP biological distribution and its flow time in circulation imprints critical parameters for cancer therapy. Numerical models advise that NP size can control its various interaction with cells, mainly with the endothelial wall of vessels of cancer *via* marginal dynamic mechanism [110]. Lastly, the surface structure of the NP can affect its cell uptake. Current studies have shown that NPs coated with sub-nanometer striations explains increased uptake compared with random surface structures [111].

Targeted NPs

Recent advances in cancer proteomics and bioinformatics referred to as a "magic bullet" by the visionary Paul Ehrlich [112] which allowed the development of targeted therapies, that act as nanocarriers which are surface functionalized with biomolecules for "active" tumour site targeting. Surface ligands like antibodies, aptamers, peptides or small molecules which recognize the tumour-specific or tumour-associated antigens in the tumour microenvironment [113 - 116] and by this active targeting mechanism highly specific interactions with tumour tissues or with cell surface antigens occur to enhance cellular uptake and increase retention within tumours. Conjugation approaches have been developed to control the amount of targeting ligands on the surface of the NPs. The two means of approach for receptor-mediated targeting are firstly by targeting the tumour microenvironment, including the extracellular matrix or surface receptors on tumour blood vessel endothelial cells (Fig. **11**), and it is commonly very effective for the delivery of immune induction or anti-angiogenesis molecules. Secondly, target tumour cell surface receptors are used for intracellular delivery (Fig. **12**) of anticancer agents or signal-pathway inhibitors. Transmembrane tumour antigen on the extracellular membrane are approached by nano-carriers through receptor led endocytosis and cancer cell uptake, hence delivering therapeutic drug load extracellularly and is quiet efficient too.

Active Targeting of Cancer Cells

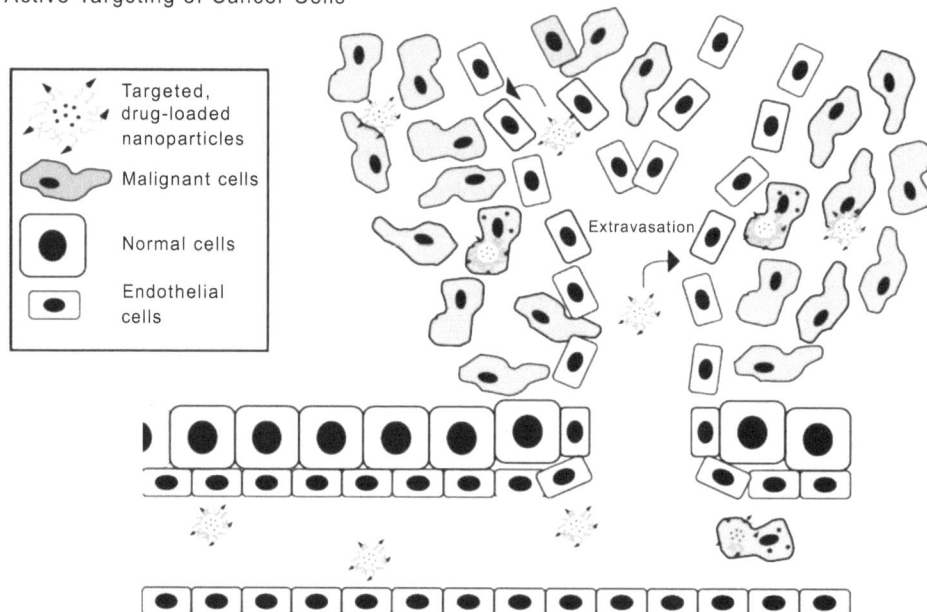

Fig. (11). Schematic diagram of active targeting of functionalized NPs to cancer cells. Targeting ligands on the surface of NPs are able to bind to receptors on malignant cells, causing local drug delivery or uptake through receptor mediated endocytosis [39].

Cancer metastasis treatment still remains a challenge even after the development of so many approaches and therapies. Targeted NP enclosing cytotoxic drug doxorubicin using integral receptor has shown few benefits in the treatment of primary and metastatic sites of human renal and pancreatic carcinoma mouse xenograft models [117]. Targeted nano particles used in the treatment of primary tumour and nodal metastasis in liver had shown effect like increased drug accumulation at tumour site and reduction in the tumour weight. Aptamer functionalized NP was developed by Alexis *et al* [118] for controlled drug released for multiple cancer types. Aptamers bind to specific targets and have various clinical uses as they have good target affinity and specificity. In a clinical evaluation np bound aptamer used as targeting ligand had led to total reduction in tumour size in human prostatic carcinoma xenograft mice model [115, 119] improving the survival and extending upto 3 months in comparison with controls. Subsequently, they also reported a new strategical formulation targeted NPs that was tested under *in vivo* [120].

Active Targeting of Angiogenic Endothelial Cells

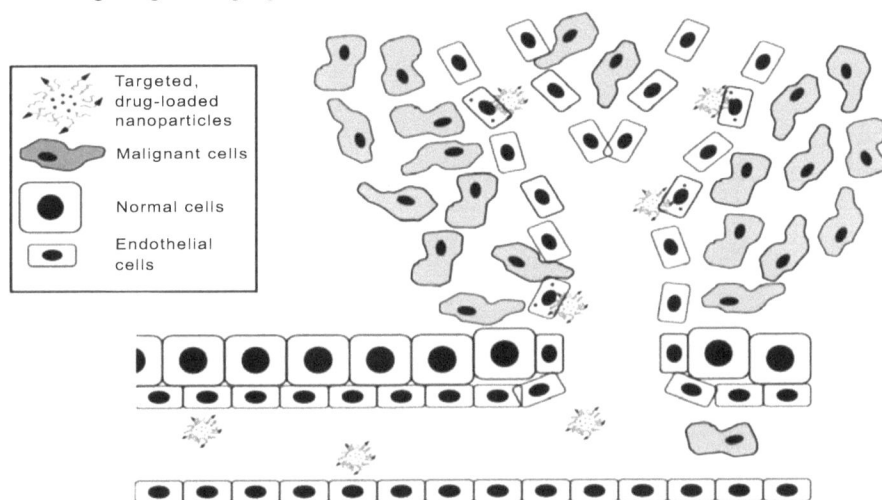

Fig. (12). Schematic diagram of active targeting of functionalized NPs to the endothelial wall. Targeting ligands on the surface of NPs are able to bind to receptors on endothelial cells or basement membrane matrix, causing local drug delivery on the endothelial wall for anti- angiogenesis therapy [39].

TARGETING EFFLUX-PUMP-MEDIATED RESISTANCE

Multi drug resistance (MDR) is the biggest problem encountered in clinical practices which reduces the efficacy of the cancer therapy [121, 122]. The resistance is targeting efflux-pump-mediated which is caused by cancer cells. The mechanism of the MDR is by physiological barriers from non-cellular based mechanisms and also by changes in cellular biochemical mechanism. Non-cellular MDR is due to poor tumour vascularization which prevents the drug to reach the tumour site and hence causing resistance. In cellular MDR the resistance occurs due to change in the specific enzymes which are related to metabolism of the drug used hence reducing the apoptosis, causing cellular repair mutation of target and increasing the efflux of the drug from tumour cells. For example, P-glycoprotein is a discovered drug efflux pump that causes active efflux of drugs from tumour cells emerging as a possible cause of cellular MDR [123, 124]. P-gp is a 170 kDa transmembrane glycoprotein responsible for efflux pump (removes the drug out of the cells actively) inherited by MDR 1 gene. To combat this inhibitors of AbC transporters are developed as a class of anticancer drugs but were not helpful [125]. To overcome this resistance NP based drugs were developed were helpful since allow selective tumour cell accumulation without any systemic toxicity since they directly enter the cells *via* endocytosis (Fig. **13**). Using a proper NP design the drug can be protected from the harsh environment of the GIT acidic pH enzymes and various degrading agents like nucleases for example. The tumour cells can be targeted and the drug can be specifically accumulated without encountering any change for example doxorubicin loaded poly-alkyl cyanoacrylate (PACA) NPs are able to penetrate cells without being recognized by P- gp [126, 127] using PACA NPs, it has been explained that the MDR ofP388 leukemia cells in culture were partially overcome. PEG-coated PACA NPs were prepared from a poly- PEG-cyanoacrylateco -hexadecyl cyanoacrylate co-polymer [127]. Drug administration in the form of PEG coated PACA nanoparticle study was conducted on murine cancer models showed better accumulation of the drug in the tumour cells [128]. Additionally, Schluep *et al* [129] showed that IT-101 administered systemically in mice can overcome P-gp resistance in mouse tumour xenograft. It is in regular consistent with the hypothesis that polymeric drug conjugates are able to overcome certain kinds of MDR (Fig. **13**).

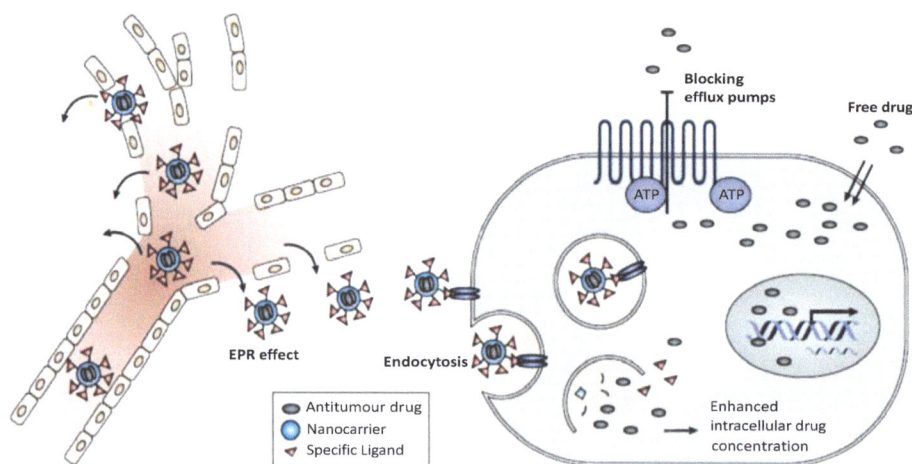

Fig. (13). Showing surface efflux pump MDR can be reduced by NP. Efflux- pump mediated resistance leading to increased elimination of drug entering the cell is shown with the drugs that inhibit the efflux pump which have low success till now. Also NPs which increase the permeability and retain in the blood vessels of tumours are shown to target surface receptors and enter the tumour site through endocytosis and load the drug. NPs allow high drug concentrations in the tumour cells owing to its property thus over coming efflux-pump mediated drug resistance [130].

The strategies concerned with use of targeted NPs have an advantage of their binding to cell-surface receptors which are taken and broken up by endocytosis and this mechanism has also been applied to overcome drug resistance. Folate-receptor targeted, pH-sensitive polymeric micelles containing doxorubicin [131], transferrin-conjugated paclitaxel NPs [132] and oxaliplatin transferrin-ligated liposomes [133] show a great anti-tumour activity than the respective free drugs in drug- resistant mouse models. Studies conducted reveals that various NPs which contain micro molecular drugs and targeted moieties are superior to non-targeted NPs. But a proof has to be gathered regarding surface pump mediated resistance was bypassed by NP since the response in the patients clinically was partial [134, 135], who received the drugs before with a failure of response is quite a possibility. For example, patients who were refractory to prior taxane therapy (for example, non-small-cell lung cancer with paclitaxel/carboplatin and ovarian cancer with paclitaxel/carboplatin and paclitaxel regimens) experienced objective responses after treatments with Genexol-PM, a polymeric micelle NP containing paclitaxel, or XYoTAX (CT-2103), a PG-paclitaxel conjugate [135, 136].

CONCLUSION

Targeted NPs administered orally exhibit a large number of potential biomedical applications and known for several putative advantages for oral drug delivery, such as the protection of fragile drugs or the potential for the modification of drug pharmacokinetics. Despite of these many advantages, the oral delivery of drugs by NPs still stand challenging. To make an efficient drug delivery, NPs must possess i) have a stable absorption rate irrespective of mucous clearance, ii) easily penetrate the mucus layer, iii) must be extensively absorbed by GI epithelium, iv) should not be affected by the barriers such as blood brain barrier *etc.*, v) should not have fast metabolism / elimination by kidneys and liver, vi) should not be affected by gastric acid secretions/ pH and vii) should have minimal drug interaction. The optimization of particle size and surface properties and the targeting of specific cells by ligand grafting have been shown to enhance NP transport across the intestinal epithelium.

The main usage of Nanoparticles is their challenging properties that are improved by the use of ligands that are not being degraded in the GI tract, unlike peptidic/proteinic ligands, and are not restricted to receptors which interact only with proteins. The utilization of NPs as drug carriers promises a gradient improvement in cancer treatment. Targeted delivery can reduce the side effects systemically which must endure patients under traditional chemotherapy by ensuring that pronounced cytotoxic levels of the drugs are only present at the tumour sites. NPs have been designed to release their drug loads in response to a variety of stimuli, either those specific to the tumour microenvironment, such as acidic pH values and elevated secretion of certain enzymes (*e.g.,* matrix metalloproteinases), or external ones, such as light exposure and heating, among others.

In the past few years, NP based delivery systems also started to show promising note for cancer immunotherapy since these therapies allow the release of tumour-associated immunomodulatory agents and/or antigens to dendritic cells. In the recent technical advancements along with knowledge accumulated over the past decades, we believe that smart, targeted NPs as drug carriers will revolutionize the field of cancer chemotherapy by significantly improving both the quality of treatment and duration of patient's life. We hope to see in the near future, the development of personalized cancer therapies based on NPs with more sophisticated designs and integrations.

However, a new horizon of nanotechnology based therapies are on the emerging wave and are going to change the world of medical science. Nanotechnology is expected to play an important part in improving the management of various diseases like cancer etc. within the next decade. The medical applications for nanotechnology are enormous and could give medicine, including the treatment of cancer, an entirely new outlook.

CONFLICT OF INTEREST

The authors declares no conflict of interest, financial or otherwise.

ACKNOWLEDGEMENTS

None Declared.

REFERENCES

[1]   Schenk M, Mueller C. The mucosal immune system at the gastrointestinal barrier. Best Pract Res Clin Gastroenterol 2008; 22(3): 391-409.
        [http://dx.doi.org/10.1016/j.bpg.2007.11.002] [PMID: 18492562]

[2]   Frey A, Giannasca KT, Weltzin R, *et al.* Role of the glycocalyx in regulating access of microparticles to apical plasma membranes of intestinal epithelial cells: implications for microbial attachment and oral vaccine targeting. J Exp Med 1996; 184(3): 1045-59.
        [http://dx.doi.org/10.1084/jem.184.3.1045] [PMID: 9064322]

[3]   Yun Y, Cho YW, Park K. Nanoparticles for oral delivery: targeted nanoparticles with peptidic ligands for oral protein delivery. Adv Drug Deliv Rev 2013; 65(6): 822-32.
        [http://dx.doi.org/10.1016/j.addr.2012.10.007] [PMID: 23123292]

[4]   Plapied L, Duhem N, des Rieux A, Préat V. Fate of polymeric nanocarriers for oral drug delivery. Curr Opin Colloid Interface Sci 2011; 16(3): 228-37.
        [http://dx.doi.org/10.1016/j.cocis.2010.12.005]

[5]   Cone RA. Barrier properties of mucus. Adv Drug Deliv Rev 2009; 61(2): 75-85.
        [http://dx.doi.org/10.1016/j.addr.2008.09.008] [PMID: 19135107]

[6]   Lai SK, Wang YY, Hanes J. Mucus-penetrating nanoparticles for drug and gene delivery to mucosal tissues. Adv Drug Deliv Rev 2009; 61(2): 158-71.
        [http://dx.doi.org/10.1016/j.addr.2008.11.002] [PMID: 19133304]

[7]   Suk JS, Lai SK, Wang YY, *et al.* The penetration of fresh undiluted sputum expectorated by cystic

fibrosis patients by non-adhesive polymer nanoparticles. Biomaterials 2009; 30(13): 2591-7.
[http://dx.doi.org/10.1016/j.biomaterials.2008.12.076] [PMID: 19176245]

[8]   Tang BC, Dawson M, Lai SK, *et al.* Biodegradable polymer nanoparticles that rapidly penetrate the human mucus barrier. Proc Natl Acad Sci USA 2009; 106(46): 19268-73.
[http://dx.doi.org/10.1073/pnas.0905998106] [PMID: 19901335]

[9]   Suk JS, Lai SK, Boylan NJ, Dawson MR, Boyle MP, Hanes J. Rapid transport of muco-inert nanoparticles in cystic fibrosis sputum treated with N-acetyl cysteine. Nanomedicine (Lond) 2011; 6(2): 365-75.
[http://dx.doi.org/10.2217/nnm.10.123] [PMID: 21385138]

[10]   Yang M, Lai SK, Wang YY, *et al.* Biodegradable nanoparticles composed entirely of safe materials that rapidly penetrate human mucus. Angew Chem Int Ed Engl 2011; 50(11): 2597-600.
[http://dx.doi.org/10.1002/anie.201006849] [PMID: 21370345]

[11]   Tailford LE, Crost EH, Kavanaugh D, Juge N. Mucin glycan foraging in the human gut microbiome. Front Genet 2015; 6: 81-7.
[http://dx.doi.org/10.3389/fgene.2015.00081] [PMID: 25852737]

[12]   Corfield AP. Mucins: a biologically relevant glycan barrier in mucosal protection. Biochim Biophys Acta 2015; 1850(1): 236-52.
[http://dx.doi.org/10.1016/j.bbagen.2014.05.003] [PMID: 24821013]

[13]   Ensign LM, Cone R, Hanes J. Oral drug delivery with polymeric nanoparticles: the gastrointestinal mucus barriers. Adv Drug Deliv Rev 2012; 64(6): 557-70.
[http://dx.doi.org/10.1016/j.addr.2011.12.009] [PMID: 22212900]

[14]   Cone R. In: Mestecky J, Lamm ME, Ogra PL, Strober W, Bienenstock J, McGhee JR, Mayer L, editors. Mucosal immunology. London Academic Press 2005; pp. 49-72.

[15]   Corfield AP, Carroll D, Myerscough N, Probert CS. Mucins in the gastrointestinal tract in health and disease. Front Biosci 2001; 6(10): D1321-57.
[http://dx.doi.org/10.2741/A684] [PMID: 11578958]

[16]   Linden SK, Sutton P, Karlsson NG, Korolik V, McGuckin MA. Mucins in the mucosal barrier to infection. Mucosal Immunol 2008; 1(3): 183-97.
[http://dx.doi.org/10.1038/mi.2008.5] [PMID: 19079178]

[17]   Lang T, Klasson S, Larsson E, Johansson ME, Hansson GC, Samuelsson T. Searching the evolutionary origin of epithelial mucus protein components-mucins and FCGBP 2016.
[http://dx.doi.org/10.1093/molbev/msw066]

[18]   MacAdam A. The effect of gastrointestinal mucus on drug absorption. Adv Drug Deliv Rev 1993; 11(3): 201-20.
[http://dx.doi.org/10.1016/0169-409X(93)90010-2]

[19]   Jia L. Global governmental investment in nanotechnologies. Curr Nanosci 2005; 1(3): 263-6.
[http://dx.doi.org/10.2174/157341305774642957] [PMID: 19865495]

[20]   Nikalje AP. Nanotechnology and its Applications in Medicine. Med Chem 2015; 2015
[http://dx.doi.org/10.4172/2161-0444.1000247]

[21]   Wilczewska AZ, Niemirowicz K, Markiewicz KH, Car H. Nanoparticles as drug delivery systems. Pharmacol Rep 2012; 64(5): 1020-37.
[http://dx.doi.org/10.1016/S1734-1140(12)70901-5] [PMID: 23238461]

[22]   des Rieux A, Fievez V, Garinot M, Schneider YJ, Préat V. Nanoparticles as potential oral delivery systems of proteins and vaccines: a mechanistic approach. J Control Release 2006; 116(1): 1-27.
[http://dx.doi.org/10.1016/j.jconrel.2006.08.013] [PMID: 17050027]

[23]   Lasoń E, Sikora E, Ogonowski J. Influence of process parameters on properties of Nanostructured Lipid Carriers (NLC) formulation. Acta Biochim Pol 2013; 60(4): 773-7.

[PMID: 24432330]

[24]   Kumar BG. Advancements in Novel Drug Delivery Systems and Opportunities for Indian Pharmaceutical companies. J Pharm Nanotechnol 2015; 4: 32-5.

[25]   Anand P, Kunnumakkara AB, Sundaram C, *et al.* Cancer is a preventable disease that requires major lifestyle changes. Pharm Res 2008; 25(9): 2097-116.
       [http://dx.doi.org/10.1007/s11095-008-9661-9] [PMID: 18626751]

[26]   International Agency for Research on Cancer. World cancer report 2014.

[27]   World Health Organization. Global Battle against Cancer Won't Be Won with Treatment Alone Effective Prevention Measures Urgently Needed to Prevent Cancer Crisis 2014.

[28]   Lee KS, Chung HC, Im SA, *et al.* Multicenter phase II trial of Genexol-PM, a Cremophor-free, polymeric micelle formulation of paclitaxel, in patients with metastatic breast cancer. Breast Cancer Res Treat 2008; 108(2): 241-50.
       [http://dx.doi.org/10.1007/s10549-007-9591-y] [PMID: 17476588]

[29]   Walko CM, McLeod H. Pharmacogenomic progress in individualized dosing of key drugs for cancer patients. Nat Clin Pract Oncol 2009; 6(3): 153-62.
       [http://dx.doi.org/10.1038/ncponc1303] [PMID: 19174777]

[30]   Bharali DJ, Mousa SA. Emerging nanomedicines for early cancer detection and improved treatment: current perspective and future promise. Pharmacol Ther 2010; 128(2): 324-35.
       [http://dx.doi.org/10.1016/j.pharmthera.2010.07.007] [PMID: 20705093]

[31]   Sun T, Zhang YS, Pang B, Hyun DC, Yang M, Xia Y. Engineered nanoparticles for drug delivery in cancer therapy 2014.

[32]   Whitesides GM. The 'right' size in nanobiotechnology. Nat Biotechnol 2003; 21(10): 1161-5.
       [http://dx.doi.org/10.1038/nbt872] [PMID: 14520400]

[33]   LaVan DA, McGuire T, Langer R. Small-scale systems for *in vivo* drug delivery. Nat Biotechnol 2003; 21(10): 1184-91.
       [http://dx.doi.org/10.1038/nbt876] [PMID: 14520404]

[34]   Farokhzad OC, Karp JM, Langer R. Nanoparticle-aptamer bioconjugates for cancer targeting. Expert Opin Drug Deliv 2006; 3(3): 311-24.
       [http://dx.doi.org/10.1517/17425247.3.3.311] [PMID: 16640493]

[35]   Farokhzad OC, Langer R. Impact of nanotechnology on drug delivery. ACS Nano 2009; 3(1): 16-20.
       [http://dx.doi.org/10.1021/nn900002m] [PMID: 19206243]

[36]   Li J, Xue S, Mao ZW. Nanoparticle delivery systems for siRNA-based therapeutics. J Mater Chem B Mater Biol Med 2016; 4(41): 6620-39.
       [http://dx.doi.org/10.1039/C6TB01462C]

[37]   Thomas CR, Ferris DP, Lee JH, *et al.* Noninvasive remote-controlled release of drug molecules *in vitro* using magnetic actuation of mechanized nanoparticles. J Am Chem Soc 2010; 132(31): 10623-5.
       [http://dx.doi.org/10.1021/ja1022267] [PMID: 20681678]

[38]   Lobatto ME, Fuster V, Fayad ZA, Mulder WJ. Perspectives and opportunities for nanomedicine in the management of atherosclerosis. Nat Rev Drug Discov 2011; 10(11): 835-52.
       [http://dx.doi.org/10.1038/nrd3578] [PMID: 22015921]

[39]   Alexis F, Pridgen EM, Langer R, Farokhzad OC. Nanoparticle technologies for cancer therapy. Handb Exp Pharmacol 2010; 197(197): 55-86.
       [http://dx.doi.org/10.1007/978-3-642-00477-3_2] [PMID: 20217526]

[40]   Couvreur P. Nanoparticles in drug delivery: past, present and future. Adv Drug Deliv Rev 2013; 65(1): 21-3.
       [http://dx.doi.org/10.1016/j.addr.2012.04.010] [PMID: 22580334]

[41] Bao G, Mitragotri S, Tong S. Multifunctional nanoparticles for drug delivery and molecular imaging. Annu Rev Biomed Eng 2013; 15: 253-82.
[http://dx.doi.org/10.1146/annurev-bioeng-071812-152409] [PMID: 23642243]

[42] Langer R, Folkman J. Polymers for the sustained release of proteins and other macromolecules. Nature 1976; 263(5580): 797-800.
[http://dx.doi.org/10.1038/263797a0] [PMID: 995197]

[43] Gref R, Minamitake Y, Peracchia MT, Trubetskoy V, Torchilin V, Langer R. Biodegradable long-circulating polymeric nanospheres 1994.
[http://dx.doi.org/10.1126/science.8128245]

[44] Jokerst JV, Lobovkina T, Zare RN, Gambhir SS. Nanoparticle PEGylation for imaging and therapy. Nanomedicine (Lond) 2011; 6(4): 715-28.
[http://dx.doi.org/10.2217/nnm.11.19] [PMID: 21718180]

[45] Tejada-Berges T, Granai CO, Gordinier M, Gajewski W. Caelyx/Doxil for the treatment of metastatic ovarian and breast cancer. Expert Rev Anticancer Ther 2002; 2(2): 143-50.
[http://dx.doi.org/10.1586/14737140.2.2.143] [PMID: 12113236]

[46] Sercombe L, Veerati T, Moheimani F, Wu SY, Sood AK, Hua S. Advances and challenges of liposome assisted drug delivery. Front Pharmacol 2015; 6: 286-92.
[http://dx.doi.org/10.3389/fphar.2015.00286] [PMID: 26648870]

[47] http://www.clinicaltrials.gov

[48] Pridgen EM, Langer R, Farokhzad OC. Biodegradable, polymeric nanoparticle delivery systems for cancer therapy. Nanomedicine (Lond) 2007; 2(5): 669-80.
[http://dx.doi.org/10.2217/17435889.2.5.669] [PMID: 17976029]

[49] Kim J, Wilson DR, Zamboni CG, Green JJ. Targeted polymeric nanoparticles for cancer gene therapy. J Drug Target 2015; 23(7-8): 627-41.
[http://dx.doi.org/10.3109/1061186X.2015.1048519] [PMID: 26061296]

[50] Torchilin VP. Recent advances with liposomes as pharmaceutical carriers. Nat Rev Drug Discov 2005; 4(2): 145-60.
[http://dx.doi.org/10.1038/nrd1632] [PMID: 15688077]

[51] Assanhou AG, Li W, Zhang L, *et al.* Reversal of multidrug resistance by co-delivery of paclitaxel and lonidamine using a TPGS and hyaluronic acid dual-functionalized liposome for cancer treatment. Biomaterials 2015; 73: 284-95.
[http://dx.doi.org/10.1016/j.biomaterials.2015.09.022] [PMID: 26426537]

[52] Fan H. Nanocrystal-micelle: synthesis, self-assembly and application. Chem Commun (Camb) 2008; 12(12): 1383-94.
[http://dx.doi.org/10.1039/B711251N] [PMID: 18338033]

[53] Matsumura Y. Poly (amino acid) micelle nanocarriers in preclinical and clinical studies. Adv Drug Deliv Rev 2008; 60(8): 899-914.
[http://dx.doi.org/10.1016/j.addr.2007.11.010] [PMID: 18406004]

[54] Xie J, Zhang X, Teng M, *et al.* Synthesis, characterization, and evaluation of mPEG-SN38 and mPEG-PLA-SN38 micelles for cancer therapy. Int J Nanomedicine 2016; 11: 1677-86.
[PMID: 27217746]

[55] Florence AT, Hussain N. Transcytosis of nanoparticle and dendrimer delivery systems: evolving vistas. Adv Drug Deliv Rev 2001; 50 (Suppl. 1): S69-89.
[http://dx.doi.org/10.1016/S0169-409X(01)00184-3] [PMID: 11576696]

[56] Najlah M, D'Emanuele A. Synthesis of dendrimers and drug-dendrimer conjugates for drug delivery. Curr Opin Drug Discov Devel 2007; 10(6): 756-67.
[PMID: 17987527]

[57]   Greco F, Vicent MJ. Polymer-drug conjugates: current status and future trends. Front Biosci 2008; 13(1): 2744-56.
[http://dx.doi.org/10.2741/2882] [PMID: 17981750]

[58]   Murakami T, Tsuchida K. Recent advances in inorganic nanoparticle-based drug delivery systems. Mini Rev Med Chem 2008; 8(2): 175-83.
[http://dx.doi.org/10.2174/138955708783498078] [PMID: 18289101]

[59]   Sirelkhatim A, Mahmud S, Seeni A, Kaus NH. Preferential cytotoxicity of ZnO nanoparticle towards cervical cancer cells induced by ROS-mediated apoptosis and cell cycle arrest for cancer therapy. J Nanopart Res 2016; 18(8): 219.
[http://dx.doi.org/10.1007/s11051-016-3531-x]

[60]   Zhang L, Granick S. How to stabilize phospholipid liposomes (using nanoparticles). Nano Lett 2006; 6(4): 694-8.
[http://dx.doi.org/10.1021/nl052455y] [PMID: 16608266]

[61]   Bozzuto G, Molinari A. Liposomes as nanomedical devices. Int J Nanomedicine 2015; 10: 975-99.
[http://dx.doi.org/10.2147/IJN.S68861] [PMID: 25678787]

[62]   Qiu L, Jing N, Jin Y. Preparation and *in vitro* evaluation of liposomal chloroquine diphosphate loaded by a transmembrane pH-gradient method. Int J Pharm 2008; 361(1-2): 56-63.
[http://dx.doi.org/10.1016/j.ijpharm.2008.05.010] [PMID: 18573626]

[63]   Hoffman AS. The origins and evolution of "controlled" drug delivery systems. J Control Release 2008; 132(3): 153-63.
[http://dx.doi.org/10.1016/j.jconrel.2008.08.012] [PMID: 18817820]

[64]   Riggio C, Pagni E, Raffa V, Cuschieri A. Nano-oncology: clinical application for cancer therapy and future perspectives. J of Nanomat 2011; 2011: 17-21.

[65]   Couvreur P, Kante B, Roland M, Speiser P. Adsorption of antineoplastic drugs to polyalkylcyanoacrylate nanoparticles and their release in calf serum. J Pharm Sci 1979; 68(12): 1521-4.
[http://dx.doi.org/10.1002/jps.2600681215] [PMID: 529043]

[66]   Ulbrich K, Holá K, Šubr V, Bakandritsos A, Tuček J, Zbořil R. Targeted drug delivery with polymers and magnetic nanoparticles: covalent and noncovalent approaches, release control, and clinical studies. Chem Rev 2016; 116(9): 5338-431.
[http://dx.doi.org/10.1021/acs.chemrev.5b00589] [PMID: 27109701]

[67]   Gref R, Lück M, Quellec P, et al. 'Stealth' corona-core nanoparticles surface modified by polyethylene glycol (PEG): influences of the corona (PEG chain length and surface density) and of the core composition on phagocytic uptake and plasma protein adsorption. Colloids Surf B Biointerfaces 2000; 18(3-4): 301-13.
[http://dx.doi.org/10.1016/S0927-7765(99)00156-3] [PMID: 10915952]

[68]   Vasey PA, Kaye SB, Morrison R, et al. Cancer Research Campaign Phase I/II Committee. Phase I clinical and pharmacokinetic study of PK1 [N-(2-hydroxypropyl)methacrylamide copolymer doxorubicin]: first member of a new class of chemotherapeutic agents-drug-polymer conjugates. Clin Cancer Res 1999; 5(1): 83-94.
[PMID: 9918206]

[69]   Sood P, Thurmond KB II, Jacob JE, et al. Synthesis and characterization of AP5346, a novel polymer-linked diaminocyclohexyl platinum chemotherapeutic agent. Bioconjug Chem 2006; 17(5): 1270-9.
[http://dx.doi.org/10.1021/bc0600517] [PMID: 16984138]

[70]   Rice JR, Gerberich JL, Nowotnik DP, Howell SB. Preclinical efficacy and pharmacokinetics of AP5346, a novel diaminocyclohexane-platinum tumor-targeting drug delivery system. Clin Cancer Res 2006; 12(7 Pt 1): 2248-54.
[http://dx.doi.org/10.1158/1078-0432.CCR-05-2169] [PMID: 16609041]

[71]   Doppalapudi S, Jain A, Domb AJ, Khan W. Biodegradable polymers for targeted delivery of anti-cancer drugs. Expert Opin Drug Deliv 2016; 13(6): 891-909.
[PMID: 26983898]

[72]   Li C. Poly(L-glutamic acid)--anticancer drug conjugates. Adv Drug Deliv Rev 2002; 54(5): 695-713.
[http://dx.doi.org/10.1016/S0169-409X(02)00045-5] [PMID: 12204599]

[73]   Homsi J, Simon GR, Garrett CR, *et al.* Phase I trial of poly-L-glutamate camptothecin (CT-2106) administered weekly in patients with advanced solid malignancies. Clin Cancer Res 2007; 13(19): 5855-61.
[http://dx.doi.org/10.1158/1078-0432.CCR-06-2821] [PMID: 17908979]

[74]   Singer JW, Baker B, de Vries P, Kumar A, Shaffer S, Vawter E, *et al.* Poly-(l)-glutamic acid-paclitaxel (CT-2103)[XYOTAX™], a biodegradable polymeric drug conjugate. InPolymer drugs in the clinical stage. Adv Exp Med Biol 2003; 519: 81-99.
[http://dx.doi.org/10.1007/0-306-47932-X_6] [PMID: 12675210]

[75]   Boddy AV, Plummer ER, Todd R, *et al.* A phase I and pharmacokinetic study of paclitaxel poliglumex (XYOTAX), investigating both 3-weekly and 2-weekly schedules. Clin Cancer Res 2005; 11(21): 7834-40.
[http://dx.doi.org/10.1158/1078-0432.CCR-05-0803] [PMID: 16278406]

[76]   Oerlemans C, Bult W, Bos M, Storm G, Nijsen JF, Hennink WE. Polymeric micelles in anticancer therapy: targeting, imaging and triggered release. Pharm Res 2010; 27(12): 2569-89.
[http://dx.doi.org/10.1007/s11095-010-0233-4] [PMID: 20725771]

[77]   Aliabadi HM, Shahin M, Brocks DR, Lavasanifar A. Disposition of drugs in block copolymer micelle delivery systems: from discovery to recovery. Clin Pharmacokinet 2008; 47(10): 619-34.
[http://dx.doi.org/10.2165/00003088-200847100-00001] [PMID: 18783294]

[78]   Lee KS, Chung HC, Im SA, *et al.* Multicenter phase II trial of Genexol-PM, a Cremophor-free, polymeric micelle formulation of paclitaxel, in patients with metastatic breast cancer. Breast Cancer Res Treat 2008; 108(2): 241-50.
[http://dx.doi.org/10.1007/s10549-007-9591-y] [PMID: 17476588]

[79]   Uchino H, Matsumura Y, Negishi T, *et al.* Cisplatin-incorporating polymeric micelles (NC-6004) can reduce nephrotoxicity and neurotoxicity of cisplatin in rats. Br J Cancer 2005; 93(6): 678-87.
[http://dx.doi.org/10.1038/sj.bjc.6602772] [PMID: 16222314]

[80]   Matsumura Y, Hamaguchi T, Ura T, *et al.* Phase I clinical trial and pharmacokinetic evaluation of NK911, a micelle-encapsulated doxorubicin. Br J Cancer 2004; 91(10): 1775-81.
[http://dx.doi.org/10.1038/sj.bjc.6602204] [PMID: 15477860]

[81]   Kim SC, Kim DW, Shim YH, *et al. In vivo* evaluation of polymeric micellar paclitaxel formulation: toxicity and efficacy. J Control Release 2001; 72(1-3): 191-202.
[http://dx.doi.org/10.1016/S0168-3659(01)00275-9] [PMID: 11389998]

[82]   Krishnamurthy S, Ng VW, Gao S, Tan MH, Yang YY. Phenformin-loaded polymeric micelles for targeting both cancer cells and cancer stem cells *in vitro* and *in vivo.* Biomaterials 2014; 35(33): 9177-86.
[http://dx.doi.org/10.1016/j.biomaterials.2014.07.018] [PMID: 25106770]

[83]   Matsumura Y, Kataoka K. Preclinical and clinical studies of anticancer agent-incorporating polymer micelles. Cancer Sci 2009; 100(4): 572-9.
[http://dx.doi.org/10.1111/j.1349-7006.2009.01103.x] [PMID: 19462526]

[84]   Discher BM, Won YY, Ege DS, *et al.* Polymersomes: tough vesicles made from diblock copolymers. Science 1999; 284(5417): 1143-6.
[http://dx.doi.org/10.1126/science.284.5417.1143] [PMID: 10325219]

[85]   Ahmed F, Pakunlu RI, Srinivas G, *et al.* Shrinkage of a rapidly growing tumor by drug-loaded polymersomes: pH-triggered release through copolymer degradation. Mol Pharm 2006; 3(3): 340-50.

[http://dx.doi.org/10.1021/mp050103u] [PMID: 16749866]

[86]   Gradishar WJ. Albumin-bound paclitaxel: a next-generation taxane. Expert Opin Pharmacother 2006; 7(8): 1041-53.
[http://dx.doi.org/10.1517/14656566.7.8.1041] [PMID: 16722814]

[87]   Nyman DW, Campbell KJ, Hersh E, *et al.* Phase I and pharmacokinetics trial of ABI-007, a novel nanoparticle formulation of paclitaxel in patients with advanced nonhematologic malignancies. J Clin Oncol 2005; 23(31): 7785-93.
[http://dx.doi.org/10.1200/JCO.2004.00.6148] [PMID: 16258082]

[88]   Desai N, Trieu V, Yao Z, *et al.* Increased antitumor activity, intratumor paclitaxel concentrations, and endothelial cell transport of cremophor-free, albumin-bound paclitaxel, ABI-007, compared with cremophor-based paclitaxel. Clin Cancer Res 2006; 12(4): 1317-24.
[http://dx.doi.org/10.1158/1078-0432.CCR-05-1634] [PMID: 16489089]

[89]   Lee CC, MacKay JA, Fréchet JM, Szoka FC. Designing dendrimers for biological applications. Nat Biotechnol 2005; 23(12): 1517-26.
[http://dx.doi.org/10.1038/nbt1171] [PMID: 16333296]

[90]   Peer D, Karp JM, Hong S, Farokhzad OC, Margalit R, Langer R. Nanocarriers as an emerging platform for cancer therapy. Nat Nanotechnol 2007; 2(12): 751-60.
[http://dx.doi.org/10.1038/nnano.2007.387] [PMID: 18654426]

[91]   Kukowska-Latallo JF, Candido KA, Cao Z, *et al.* Nanoparticle targeting of anticancer drug improves therapeutic response in animal model of human epithelial cancer. Cancer Res 2005; 65(12): 5317-24.
[http://dx.doi.org/10.1158/0008-5472.CAN-04-3921] [PMID: 15958579]

[92]   Myc A, Douce TB, Ahuja N, *et al.* Preclinical antitumor efficacy evaluation of dendrimer-based methotrexate conjugates. Anticancer Drugs 2008; 19(2): 143-9.
[http://dx.doi.org/10.1097/CAD.0b013e3282f28842] [PMID: 18176110]

[93]   Quintana A, Raczka E, Piehler L, *et al.* Design and function of a dendrimer-based therapeutic nanodevice targeted to tumor cells through the folate receptor. Pharm Res 2002; 19(9): 1310-6.
[http://dx.doi.org/10.1023/A:1020398624602] [PMID: 12403067]

[94]   Bartlett DW, Su H, Hildebrandt IJ, Weber WA, Davis ME. Impact of tumor-specific targeting on the biodistribution and efficacy of siRNA nanoparticles measured by multimodality *in vivo* imaging. Proc Natl Acad Sci USA 2007; 104(39): 15549-54.
[http://dx.doi.org/10.1073/pnas.0707461104] [PMID: 17875985]

[95]   Davis ME. The first targeted delivery of siRNA in humans *via* a self-assembling, cyclodextrin polymer-based nanoparticle: from concept to clinic. Mol Pharm 2009; 6(3): 659-68.
[http://dx.doi.org/10.1021/mp900015y] [PMID: 19267452]

[96]   Turney TW, Duriska MB, Jayaratne V, *et al.* Formation of zinc-containing nanoparticles from Zn^{2+} ions in cell culture media: implications for the nanotoxicology of ZnO. Chem Res Toxicol 2012; 25(10): 2057-66.
[http://dx.doi.org/10.1021/tx300241q] [PMID: 22978249]

[97]   Bisht G, Rayamajhi S. ZnO Nanoparticles: A Promising Anticancer Agent. Nanobiomedicine 2016; 3: 9.
[http://dx.doi.org/10.5772/63437]

[98]   Shen C, James SA, de Jonge MD, Turney TW, Wright PF, Feltis BN. Relating cytotoxicity, zinc ions, and reactive oxygen in ZnO nanoparticle-exposed human immune cells. Toxicol Sci 2013; 136(1): 120-30.
[http://dx.doi.org/10.1093/toxsci/kft187] [PMID: 23997113]

[99]   Johannsen M, Gneveckow U, Thiesen B, *et al.* Thermotherapy of prostate cancer using magnetic nanoparticles: feasibility, imaging, and three-dimensional temperature distribution. Eur Urol 2007; 52(6): 1653-61.

[http://dx.doi.org/10.1016/j.eururo.2006.11.023] [PMID: 17125906]

[100] Thevenot P, Cho J, Wavhal D, Timmons RB, Tang L. Surface chemistry influences cancer killing effect of TiO2 nanoparticles. Nanomedicine (Lond) 2008; 4(3): 226-36.
[http://dx.doi.org/10.1016/j.nano.2008.04.001] [PMID: 18502186]

[101] Pešić M, Podolski-Renić A, Stojković S, *et al.* Anti-cancer effects of cerium oxide nanoparticles and its intracellular redox activity. Chem Biol Interact 2015; 232: 85-93.
[http://dx.doi.org/10.1016/j.cbi.2015.03.013] [PMID: 25813935]

[102] Rao PV, Nallappan D, Madhavi K, Rahman S, Jun Wei L, Gan SH. Phytochemicals and Biogenic Metallic Nanoparticles as Anticancer Agents. Oxid Med Cell Longev 2016; 2016: 3685671.
[http://dx.doi.org/10.1155/2016/3685671] [PMID: 27057273]

[103] Chambers AF, Groom AC, MacDonald IC. Dissemination and growth of cancer cells in metastatic sites. Nat Rev Cancer 2002; 2(8): 563-72.
[http://dx.doi.org/10.1038/nrc865] [PMID: 12154349]

[104] Fidler IJ. The pathogenesis of cancer metastasis: the 'seed and soil' hypothesis revisited. Nat Rev Cancer 2003; 3(6): 453-8.
[http://dx.doi.org/10.1038/nrc1098] [PMID: 12778135]

[105] Sawaki A, Yamao K. Imatinib mesylate acts in metastatic or unresectable gastrointestinal stromal tumor by targeting KIT receptors--a review. Cancer Chemother Pharmacol 2004; 54(1) (Suppl. 1): S44-9.
[PMID: 15309514]

[106] Kim D, Lee ES, Oh KT, Gao ZG, Bae YH. Doxorubicin-loaded polymeric micelle overcomes multidrug resistance of cancer by double-targeting folate receptor and early endosomal pH. Small 2008; 4(11): 2043-50.
[http://dx.doi.org/10.1002/smll.200701275] [PMID: 18949788]

[107] Maeda H. The enhanced permeability and retention (EPR) effect in tumor vasculature: the key role of tumor-selective macromolecular drug targeting. Adv Enzyme Regul 2001; 41(1): 189-207.
[http://dx.doi.org/10.1016/S0065-2571(00)00013-3] [PMID: 11384745]

[108] Minko T, Kopečkova P, Pozharov V, Jensen KD, Kopeček J. The influence of cytotoxicity of macromolecules and of VEGF gene modulated vascular permeability on the enhanced permeability and retention effect in resistant solid tumors. Pharm Res 2000; 17(5): 505-14.
[http://dx.doi.org/10.1023/A:1007500412442] [PMID: 10888300]

[109] Hobbs SK, Monsky WL, Yuan F, *et al.* Regulation of transport pathways in tumor vessels: role of tumor type and microenvironment. Proc Natl Acad Sci USA 1998; 95(8): 4607-12.
[http://dx.doi.org/10.1073/pnas.95.8.4607] [PMID: 9539785]

[110] Decuzzi P, Ferrari M. Design maps for nanoparticles targeting the diseased microvasculature. Biomaterials 2008; 29(3): 377-84.
[http://dx.doi.org/10.1016/j.biomaterials.2007.09.025] [PMID: 17936897]

[111] Verma A, Uzun O, Hu Y, *et al.* Surface-structure-regulated cell-membrane penetration by monolayer-protected nanoparticles. Nat Mater 2008; 7(7): 588-95.
[http://dx.doi.org/10.1038/nmat2202] [PMID: 18500347]

[112] Strebhardt K, Ullrich A. Paul Ehrlich's magic bullet concept: 100 years of progress. Nat Rev Cancer 2008; 8(6): 473-80.
[http://dx.doi.org/10.1038/nrc2394] [PMID: 18469827]

[113] Alexis F, Pridgen E, Molnar LK, Farokhzad OC. Factors affecting the clearance and biodistribution of polymeric nanoparticles. Mol Pharm 2008; 5(4): 505-15.
[http://dx.doi.org/10.1021/mp800051m] [PMID: 18672949]

[114] Bareford LM, Swaan PW. Endocytic mechanisms for targeted drug delivery. Adv Drug Deliv Rev 2007; 59(8): 748-58.

[http://dx.doi.org/10.1016/j.addr.2007.06.008] [PMID: 17659804]

[115] Farokhzad OC, Cheng J, Teply BA, *et al.* Targeted nanoparticle-aptamer bioconjugates for cancer chemotherapy *in vivo.* Proc Natl Acad Sci USA 2006; 103(16): 6315-20.
[http://dx.doi.org/10.1073/pnas.0601755103] [PMID: 16606824]

[116] Sudimack J, Lee RJ. Targeted drug delivery *via* the folate receptor. Adv Drug Deliv Rev 2000; 41(2): 147-62.
[http://dx.doi.org/10.1016/S0169-409X(99)00062-9] [PMID: 10699311]

[117] Murphy EA, Majeti BK, Barnes LA, *et al.* Nanoparticle-mediated drug delivery to tumor vasculature suppresses metastasis. Proc Natl Acad Sci USA 2008; 105(27): 9343-8.
[http://dx.doi.org/10.1073/pnas.0803728105] [PMID: 18607000]

[118] Alexis F, Basto P, Levy-Nissenbaum E, *et al.* HER-2-targeted nanoparticle-affibody bioconjugates for cancer therapy. ChemMedChem 2008; 3(12): 1839-43.
[http://dx.doi.org/10.1002/cmdc.200800122] [PMID: 19012296]

[119] Farokhzad OC, Jon S, Khademhosseini A, Tran TN, Lavan DA, Langer R. Nanoparticle-aptamer bioconjugates: a new approach for targeting prostate cancer cells. Cancer Res 2004; 64(21): 7668-72.
[http://dx.doi.org/10.1158/0008-5472.CAN-04-2550] [PMID: 15520166]

[120] Gu F, Zhang L, Teply BA, *et al.* Precise engineering of targeted nanoparticles by using self-assembled biointegrated block copolymers. Proc Natl Acad Sci USA 2008; 105(7): 2586-91.
[http://dx.doi.org/10.1073/pnas.0711714105] [PMID: 18272481]

[121] Gottesman MM. Mechanisms of cancer drug resistance. Annu Rev Med 2002; 53(1): 615-27.
[http://dx.doi.org/10.1146/annurev.med.53.082901.103929] [PMID: 11818492]

[122] Gottesman MM, Fojo T, Bates SE. Multidrug resistance in cancer: role of ATP-dependent transporters. Nat Rev Cancer 2002; 2(1): 48-58.
[http://dx.doi.org/10.1038/nrc706] [PMID: 11902585]

[123] Modok S, Mellor HR, Callaghan R. Modulation of multidrug resistance efflux pump activity to overcome chemoresistance in cancer. Curr Opin Pharmacol 2006; 6(4): 350-4.
[http://dx.doi.org/10.1016/j.coph.2006.01.009] [PMID: 16690355]

[124] Nobili S, Landini I, Giglioni B, Mini E. Pharmacological strategies for overcoming multidrug resistance. Curr Drug Targets 2006; 7(7): 861-79.
[http://dx.doi.org/10.2174/138945006777709593] [PMID: 16842217]

[125] Thomas H, Coley HM. Overcoming multidrug resistance in cancer: an update on the clinical strategy of inhibiting p-glycoprotein. Cancer Control 2003; 10(2): 159-65.

[126] Pepin X, Attali L, Domrault C, *et al.* On the use of ion-pair chromatography to elucidate doxorubicin release mechanism from polyalkylcyanoacrylate nanoparticles at the cellular level. J Chromatogr B Biomed Sci Appl 1997; 702(1-2): 181-91.
[http://dx.doi.org/10.1016/S0378-4347(97)00362-9] [PMID: 9449570]

[127] Vauthier C, Dubernet C, Chauvierre C, Brigger I, Couvreur P. Drug delivery to resistant tumors: the potential of poly(alkyl cyanoacrylate) nanoparticles. J Control Release 2003; 93(2): 151-60.
[http://dx.doi.org/10.1016/j.jconrel.2003.08.005] [PMID: 14636721]

[128] Peracchia MT, Fattal E, Desmaële D, *et al.* Stealth PEGylated polycyanoacrylate nanoparticles for intravenous administration and splenic targeting. J Control Release 1999; 60(1): 121-8.
[http://dx.doi.org/10.1016/S0168-3659(99)00063-2] [PMID: 10370176]

[129] Schluep T, Hwang J, Cheng J, *et al.* Preclinical efficacy of the camptothecin-polymer conjugate IT-101 in multiple cancer models. Clin Cancer Res 2006; 12(5): 1606-14.
[http://dx.doi.org/10.1158/1078-0432.CCR-05-1566] [PMID: 16533788]

[130] Davis ME, Chen ZG, Shin DM. Nanoparticle therapeutics: an emerging treatment modality for cancer. Nat Rev Drug Discov 2008; 7(9): 771-82.

[http://dx.doi.org/10.1038/nrd2614] [PMID: 18758474]

[131] Lee ES, Na K, Bae YH. Doxorubicin loaded pH-sensitive polymeric micelles for reversal of resistant MCF-7 tumor. J Control Release 2005; 103(2): 405-18.
[http://dx.doi.org/10.1016/j.jconrel.2004.12.018] [PMID: 15763623]

[132] Sahoo SK, Ma W, Labhasetwar V. Efficacy of transferrin-conjugated paclitaxel-loaded nanoparticles in a murine model of prostate cancer. Int J Cancer 2004; 112(2): 335-40.
[http://dx.doi.org/10.1002/ijc.20405] [PMID: 15352049]

[133] Suzuki R, Takizawa T, Kuwata Y, *et al.* Effective anti-tumor activity of oxaliplatin encapsulated in transferrin-PEG-liposome. Int J Pharm 2008; 346(1-2): 143-50.
[http://dx.doi.org/10.1016/j.ijpharm.2007.06.010] [PMID: 17640835]

[134] Lee KS, Chung HC, *et al.* Multicenter phase II study of a cremophor-free polymeric micelle-formulated paclitaxel in patients (pts) with metastatic breast cancer (MBC). InASCO Annual Meeting Proceedings 2006 Jun; 24 (18) suppl: p. 10520).

[135] Nemunaitis J, Cunningham C, Senzer N, *et al.* Phase I study of CT-2103, a polymer-conjugated paclitaxel, and carboplatin in patients with advanced solid tumors. Cancer Invest 2005; 23(8): 671-6.
[http://dx.doi.org/10.1080/07357900500359935] [PMID: 16377585]

[136] Kim TY, Kim DW, Chung JY, *et al.* Phase I and pharmacokinetic study of Genexol-PM, a cremophor-free, polymeric micelle-formulated paclitaxel, in patients with advanced malignancies. Clin Cancer Res 2004; 10(11): 3708-16.
[http://dx.doi.org/10.1158/1078-0432.CCR-03-0655] [PMID: 15173077]

SUBJECT INDEX

.

www.ingramcontent.com/pod-product-compliance
Lightning Source LLC
Chambersburg PA
CBHW041728210326
41598CB00008B/812